TIRED– SO TIRED!

AND THE YEAST CONNECTION

WILLIAM G. CROOK, M.D.

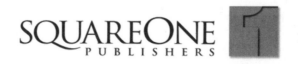

SQUAREONE
PUBLISHERS

DISCLAIMER

I've written this book to serve as a general guide for people who are tired—so tired and those who are working to help them. For obvious reasons, I cannot assume the medical or legal responsibility for having the contents of this book considered as a prescription for anyone.

To conquer and overcome your health problems, you'll need assistance from a knowledgeable and interested physician or other licensed health care professional. Accordingly, you and those who work with you must take full responsibility for the uses made of this book.

Square One Publishers

115 Herricks Road • Garden City Park, NY 11040

(516) 535-2010 • (866) 900-BOOK • www.squareonepublishers.com

Library of Congress Cataloging-in-Publication Data: 00–093515

ISBN: 978-0-7570-0063-8

Printed in China

10 9 8 7 6 5 4 3 2

Contents

To
Janet Gregory, Brenda Harris, Jan Torre

Foreword

Fatigue is no mystery. We've all experienced it and we all know what causes it. But chronic fatigue? That is a very different story, and a very puzzling story.

In simpler times, you worked hard, got a good night's rest and started the next day refreshed. That is still true for most people. But for an increasing number of us, rest, and even sleep, does not refresh, does not banish fatigue. Why? What is going on? Why is chronic fatigue increasing, and what can be done about it?

These questions are addressed at many international conferences and are the subject of many (often boring) books. The mystery of chronic fatigue continues to baffle the experts.

Enter Dr. Billy Crook; a brilliant, inquisitive, open-minded doctor of the old school who takes nothing for granted, listens carefully to his patients and his colleagues, reads the scientific literature and tempers what he learns with common sense born of long experience. He has investigated the causes of chronic fatigue for many years, and this outstanding book—which offers sufferers real hope for regaining their vigor and zest—is the result.

There are lots of doctors, and lots of books, but this book, like Dr. Crook himself, is special. Dr. Crook has learned, in his almost five decades of medical practice, that there are few simple solutions, that each patient is different—not just a little different, very different—from every other patient, and that one must be able to choose from a wide range of treatment options if one is to have any hope of success.

Tired—So Tired! provides a truly remarkable array of possible causes, and possible treatments, for chronic fatigue. No "Johnny-One-Note" is Dr. Crook! Sneak a glance at the Table of Contents and you will see what I mean. The author has really done his homework—and then some—in reviewing current research and applying the research in his medical practice to determine the causes—and the most effective treatments—for chronic fatigue.

Many years ago, in introducing Dr. Crook at a conference, I said, "The only problem with Dr. Crook is that there is only one of him. We need a Dr. Crook in every town in this country, and several dozen Dr. Crooks in every city."

I still feel that way, and after you read this book, I know you will whole-heartedly agree with me.

Bernard Rimland, Ph.D.
San Diego California

Preface

In 1992 I published a 375-page, profusely illustrated book entitled *Chronic Fatigue Syndrome and the Yeast Connection*. Here are excerpts from the Foreword of this book by Carol Jessop, M.D., Diplomate, American Board of Internal Medicine, and a faculty member of the University of California (San Francisco).

"Having worked with CFS patients for almost ten years, I believe this illness may simply represent the 10 to 15% of our species who have not adapted to the rapid and startling changes in the environment, and the subsequent changes in our internal intestinal environment.

"Since 1950 we've seen the development and overuse of antibiotics; the use of hormones and birth control pills; . . . the introduction of various chemicals and toxins into our environment; and significant changes which have occurred within our diets, leaving us food tainted with pesticides, depleted in nutritional value and loaded with sugars and dyes.

"Can we really continue to believe these incredible changes have not affected the wellbeing of some and eventually perhaps all of us? . . . Ten years ago I was very frustrated working with CFS patients because of deeply ingrained skepticism about theories such as the 'yeast connection.' However, following further research and a trial of some of these therapeutic interventions with my patients, my work has become both intellectually rewarding and fun."

In her review of *Chronic Fatigue Syndrome and the Yeast Connection*, Mary Hager, *Newsweek* health reporter said,

"Beleaguered patients will find much to cheer in Dr. Crook's new book. To start, he believes CFS is for real, that the symptoms are caused by organic changes that affect the immune system, the nervous system, the musculoskeletal system and many other parts of the body. He disagrees with conventional wisdom that CFS is 'simply a state of mind' . . .

"But even more valuable to patients may be his prescription for a hefty dose of common sense as he explores the various approaches that seem to help many patients . . . everything from diet and nutritional supplements, to new therapies on the horizon, plus, of course, his appeal that physicians and patients consider yeast infections as a potential contributor to CFS."

I made minor revisions in this book when it was reprinted in 1995, and I began working to revise it again in late 1999. But as I reviewed all of the new information that has become available in the past five years, I decided to write a new book with a different title.

Although you'll find that some of what you read in this book was included in *Chronic Fatigue Syndrome and the Yeast Connection,* two-thirds of this book is new material. Here's an even more important reason for the title change. The information and treatment program described in this book will help many weary people who have been searching for answers who do *not* meet the official criteria of CFS.

William G. Crook, M.D.

A Special Message to the Reader

If you're tired—so tired, you may have sought answers from health professionals, family members and friends. You may have been given advice of many kinds. Such as:

+ "Get more sleep."
+ "Take these vitamins."
+ "You're doing too much."
+ "See a psychiatrist."
+ "Exercise more."
+ "Try these herbal remedies."
+ "Look for a different job."
+ "Talk to your minister."

Some of this advice may be right on target. I don't know. *Although I can't promise a "quick fix" you may find many of the answers you're seeking in this book.* You can better understand what I'm talking about by comparing yourself to the proverbial overloaded camel.

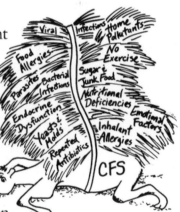

To conquer your tired feelings, to look good, feel good and enjoy life, you'll need to "unload many bundles of straw." This may take months—even a year—but then your camel will be off and running.

Acknowledgments

Beginning in the mid-1950s, I learned that sensitivities to common foods played a major role in causing fatigue, muscle aches and other symptoms in many of my pediatric patients. A few years later, the environmental pioneer, the late Theron Randolph (a Chicago internist and allergist) made me aware of the health problems caused by chemicals in the air, food, soil and water.

Then in 1979 a sick and tired adult patient that I'd been unable to help, brought me an article on candida-related health problems by Dr. C. Orian Truss. This article changed my practice and my life! Since that time, countless people, including professionals and nonprofessionals, have shared their knowledge and experiences with me, and I'm indebted to them.

Individuals who helped me gather information for this book include Nicholas Ashford, Sidney Baker, Dale Benedict, Bruce Blinzler, Robert Boxer, Renée Brehio, James Brodsky, Jean Carper, Rich Carson, Patricia Connolly, Elmer Cranton, Luke Curtis, Donald Davis, John Dommisse, Carol Englender, Mary Enig, Linda Farmer, Ann Fisk, Jorge Flechas, Charles Fox, Alan Gaby, Leo Galland, Ken Gerdes, Kathy Gibbons, Steve Gifford, Elson Haas, Rodney Harbin, Scott Heath, Ron Hoffman, Beatrice Trum Hunter, Michael Jacobson, John Jaeckle, William Jefferies, Agnes Jonas, Marjorie Jones, Paula Joyner, Kim Kenney, Chuck Knirsch, George Kroker, Charles Lapp, Richard Layton, Richard Mabray, Michael McCann, Elena McHerron, Stanley Meyerson, George Miller, Jerry Mittleman, Phillip Mosbaugh, Nick Nonas, Monica O'Kane, Becky Parks, Charles Resseger, Bernard Rimland, Sherry Rogers, Irv Rosenberg, Jean

Rowe, Todd Runestad, Beth Salmon, David Schardt, David Schlesinger, Bruce Semon, Norman Shealy, Stephen Sinatra, Jodi Smith, Peter Spencer, Jill Stansbury, Larry Stevens, Jacob Teitelbaum, Kristen Thorson, Melvyn Werbach and Ray Wunderlich.

As with my other books, I'm grateful to John Adams and the entire staff of ProtoType Graphics, Inc., Nashville, Tennessee for their skillful production services. Thanks are due also to Bill Worboys at Younger Associates who designed the cover. Special words of appreciation are again due to my daughter, Cynthia, and to Gregg Bender, for their delightful illustrations.

Last, but not least, I'm indebted to Janet Gregory, who typed and organized the manuscript and put the book together; Jan Torre who edited it; and to my secretary Brenda Harris, who helped in countless ways.

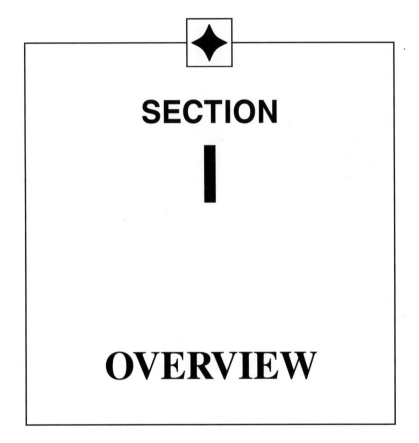

SECTION

I

OVERVIEW

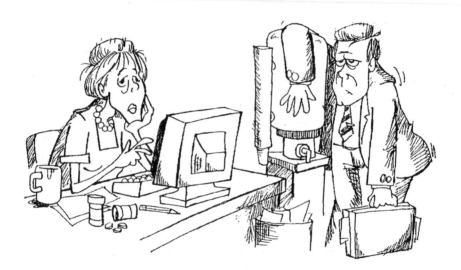

Chronic Fatigue—
An Enigma

I f you're tired, oh so tired, if your fatigue isn't relieved by rest—and you've seen many different physicians who haven't found a cause for your symptoms—you have a lot of company.

Professionals from many different disciplines, including immunology, toxicology, mycology, environmental medicine and dentistry have noted that chronic fatigue may develop from many causes. Here are some of them.

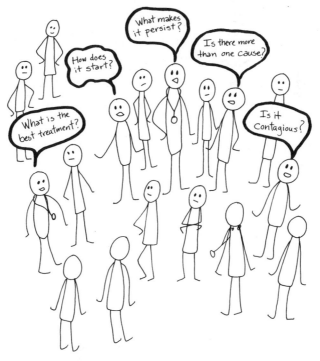

- **After a viral illness, including:** the Epstein-Barr virus, the HHV6 virus, the Coxsackie, hepatitis, influenza and other viruses.
- **After working in an airtight office building loaded with pollutants, including:** building materials which "outgas" chemical odors (formaldehyde-containing wallboard, carpet, foam rubber, paints, glues and waxes), copy papers, marking pencils, insecticides, molds in the air conditioning system, tobacco smoke, perfumes and other cosmetics, floor cleaners, and bathroom chemicals.

  Illness that develops in office workers exposed to these substances has been called the "sick building syndrome."
- **After living in a home polluted with environmental chemicals.** These include cigarette smoke, cosmetics, pesticides, laundry and bathroom chemicals, gas cooking stoves, freshly dry-cleaned clothes and many of the same pollutants found in office buildings.
- **After exposure to toxic chemicals in a factory.**
- **After living in the tropics and acquiring a parasitic infection.**
- **Living in a damp, moldy home.**
- **Following the insertion of mercury/amalgam dental fillings.**
- **Proliferation of giardia and other parasites** in your intestinal tract.

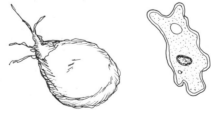

- **Consuming foods which are deficient in many essential nutrients and/or which cause allergic reactions.**
- **After taking long-term antibiotics for acne, a chronic urinary or respiratory infection or Lyme disease.**

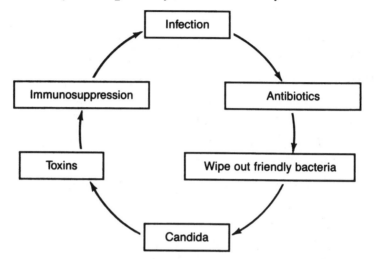

The illness cascade that then develops causes disturbances in many parts of the body.

Names, Labels and Diagnoses

Sometimes a physician can readily diagnose a medical condition. Here are some examples. A person falls while roller skating and catches his body weight on his hand. He immediately develops pain and swelling just above his wrist and an X-ray shows a fracture. The diagnosis is obvious.

A woman develops abdominal pain and nausea. Six hours after the pain starts, it moves down to the right side of her abdomen. She seeks help from a physician who examines her and finds sharply localized tenderness in the painful area. Simple laboratory tests show that her urine specimen is normal but her white blood count is elevated. A review of her menstrual history suggests that the pain and tenderness is not due to a ruptured ovarian follicle. A diagnosis of acute appendicitis seems probable.

A person has a sore throat. Tests show Group A streptococci.

But, if you're tired, tired, tired and after consulting many physicians you are told, "All of your tests are normal," what then? Does that mean that you're well, just because the tests don't show that you have a "disease"? My answer is "no."

Labeling Diseases May Not Provide the Answers We're Seeking

During the past two decades, Sidney M. Baker, M.D., a former faculty member of Yale University's School of Medicine, has said repeatedly, *"Labeling diseases isn't the way we should go."* In many presentations to professional and lay groups he says in effect,

> "When a person is tired and suffers from other chronic complaints, it's important for the physician to ask these two questions:
>
> + *"Is there something that this person needs that she is lacking?*
> + *"Is there something that she is getting too much of that contributes to her problem?*
>
> "Together, these two questions form the basis for detective work aimed at uncovering imbalances in people of all ages, with various problems. Essential lacks include:
>
> + nutrients provided by a good diet, including essential fatty acids, magnesium, B vitamins, zinc and other trace minerals
> + full spectrum light
> + clean air
> + pure water
> + love, praise, touch and other psychological nutrients
> + exercise.
>
> "The things a person should avoid as much as possible are:
>
> + pollutants in the air, food, soil and water (such as pesticides, tobacco smoke and odorous chemicals)
> + nutritionally poor foods and beverages (such as those which have been processed, packaged and loaded with sugars or contain coloring, additives and bad fats)
> + allergens
> + harmful microorganisms (including yeasts and other fungi, bacteria, viruses and parasites)"

Even before Dr. Baker made his classic comments, Emanuel Cheraskin, M.D., D.M.D., a faculty member of the University of Alabama, in an article, "The Name of the Game Is the Name," said in effect,

> "We physicians are taught to diagnose, classify and label diseases. And most of us feel if we can put a diagnostic label on each patient who comes to us we've done our duty. Then we can relax because our task becomes easy.
>
> "All we have to do then is go to our procedure book, medical library, Physician's Desk Reference (PDR) or computer and find the recommended treatment. Then we prescribe drugs, surgery or psychotherapy."[1]

And in his pioneer book *Predictive Medicine*,[2] Cheraskin said that many disabling disorders could be prevented by recognizing early signs and symptoms. He emphasized that patients with many of these disorders could be helped when they change their diets and their lifestyles.

C. Orian Truss, M.D., also commented on the "pitfall" inherent in dividing human illnesses into "diseases." In his book *The Missing Diagnosis*, he said,

> "The organs and systems of the body are so integrated . . . that to speak of disease of an individual organ is to suggest an autonomy that is undeserved. If one organ malfunctions, it is likely that there will be repercussions in most other systems."[3]

EBV, CFS and CFIDS

After over 200 people in Incline Village, Nevada, developed a lingering illness in 1984 which attracted international attention, physicians and nonphysicians began looking for "the cause" and for a "magic bullet." Initially it was thought that the Epstein-Barr Virus (EBV) was "the cause" of their health problems. Yet, tests of various sorts showed that EBV wasn't the cause. Subsequently, HHV6 and other viruses were thought to be "the causes" of the many manifestations of this chronic illness. Yet, laboratory studies failed to show that they were responsible.

In March 1988, Dr. Gary Holmes from the Division of Viral Diseases, Centers for Disease Control and Prevention, Atlanta, Georgia, and a group of scientists and clinicians published a paper entitled, "Chronic Fatigue Syndrome: A working case definition."[4] Since that time, several changes have been made in this definition.

An October 1990 publication from the National Institutes of Health, *Chronic Fatigue Syndrome, A Pamphlet for Physicians,* included a discussion of this illness. Here are excerpts.

> "Most investigators studying CFS believe that the syndrome has many possible causes . . . Preliminary research also shows a variety of immunologic disturbances in some patients. . . Several different latent viruses also appear to be reactivated in some CFS patients, although reactivation has not been shown in all patients, and it is not clear that any of these viruses are causally related to CFS or its symptoms.
>
> ". . . Most cases of CFS are sporadic: the patient does not have a close contact who had developed a similar illness . . . Although interest in this illness has grown tremendously since the mid-1980s, CFS does not appear to be a new disorder . . . Furthermore, case reports describing similar illnesses date back several centuries. . . . Many patients have a history of allergies before the onset of CFS and occasionally allergic symptoms worsen after these patients become ill. *Allergies are so prevalent in CFS patients that it is important to differentiate those symptoms that are allergy related and thus amenable to treatment . . .* (emphasis added)
>
> "In brief, no strict recipe for treating CFS exists and sometimes several different treatment approaches may have to be tried before the patient reports benefit. *Both the physician and the patient need to be open to reasonable treatment alternatives . . ."* (emphasis added)

In the late 1980s The CFIDS* Association was established with headquarters in Charlotte, North Carolina. Here are excerpts from the annual report by Marc Iverson, President of the CFIDS Association, Inc., published in the Fall 1991 issue of the nonprofit *CFIDS Chronicle*.

> "The association is governed by a large all-volunteer board of directors . . . We directly fund CFIDS research and allocate every dollar earmarked for research or advocacy . . . we publish the largest, most comprehensive CFIDS journal, the *CFIDS Chronicle* (and its supplement, The Physicians' Forum) . . . The major thrust (mission) of the CFIDS Association is educational . . .
>
> "Far too many of us, myself included, are 'battered patients' who have been victimized by conventional medical institutions, their practitioners and their rigid and arrogant doctrines. (If a condition does not fit accepted patterns and is not understood, then it is deemed to be nonexistent or of psychiatric origin.) . . . This association aggressively resists a 'medical establishment' which continues to trivialize and 'psychologize' CFIDS."

My Comments: During the past nine years I've read all of the issues of the *CFIDS Chronicle* published by the CFIDS Association. Many of the articles, letters and editorials continue to express concern about the term "chronic fatigue syndrome" because it continues to "trivialize" the disorder.

Many supporters of the CFIDS Association have said, *"We need a better diagnostic label and many labels have been suggested."* These include Myalgic Encephalomyelitis (ME), Florence Nightingale Syndrome, and some people have suggested that the disorder be named after an important researcher, dead or alive.

---

*CFIDS is the acronym for Chronic Fatigue Immune Dysfunction Syndrome.

Although there is merit in these suggestions, I concur with Drs. Baker, Cheraskin and Truss. A new "label" will not help. Scientific reports and clinical observations by physicians and scientists with impeccable credentials now demonstrate that people with CFS/CFIDS are *sick—really sick,* and need help.

Multiple causes of their sickness include nutritional deficiencies, food allergies, yeast infections, viral infections and toxins. In turn, these result in hormonal, immunologic and metabolic changes.

When these causes are carefully evaluated (as outlined by Dr. Baker) and followed by a comprehensive treatment program, many (and perhaps most) people who are *tired—so tired* will regain their health.

REFERENCES

1. Cheraskin, E., "The Name of the Game Is the Name," presented at the San Diego Medical Symposium, February 1974; *Holistic Health,* Vol. 6, 1981, pp. 73–75.

2. Cheraskin, E., *Predictive Medicine,* Pacific Press, Mt. View, CA, 1973; Keats Publishing (paperback), 1977.

3. Truss, C. O., *The Missing Diagnosis,* Box 26508, Birmingham, AL 35226, 1983/1986.

4. Holmes, G.F., et al., "Chronic Fatigue Syndrome—A working case definition," *Annals of Internal Medicine,* 108: 387–389, 1988.

More About Chronic Fatigue—And Where I'm Coming From

Depending on their background and training, professionals interested in chronic fatigue emphasize different treatment approaches and no one claims to have all the answers. Certainly, I do not. *Yet, in my pediatric, allergy and environmental medicine practice, I've found that many people with chronic fatigue, headache, muscle aches, memory loss, digestive disorders and other symptoms can be helped when they:*

✦ clean up their diet. This means eating a lot more vegetables, fruits, nuts and seeds. They can also eat some fish and lean meats. Equally important, they should avoid foods of low nutritional quality, especially sugar-laden processed foods which often contain hydrogenated or partially hydrogenated fats.

✦ get rid of chemical pollutants in their homes and work places.

✦ search for and avoid foods that cause sensitivity reactions.

✦ *take prescription and/or nonprescription antifungal medications including nystatin, Diflucan, Sporanox, Lamisil, Nizoral, amphotericin B, Lactobacillus acidophilus (and other probiotics), undecylenic acid, caprylic acid, Tanalbit, olive leaf extract, citrus seed extracts, Kyolic (or other garlic products), Kolorex, ParaCan and other substances that curb the growth of Candida albicans in the digestive tract.*

✦ take yeast-free vitamins, minerals and essential fatty acids.
✦ take vitamin B_{12}, CoQ_{10}, grape seed extract and other nutritional supplements.
✦ take thyroid supplements if they're needed.
✦ receive psychological support.

Because of my success in treating and helping many patients using this program, I've emphasized the "yeast connection" to chronic fatigue. I fully realize that I may be like one of the six blind men of Indostan who went to see the elephant.

As you'll see when you read John Godfrey Saxe's classic poem, each blind man described the elephant according to what he had seen and each blind man had a different story.

In this book I describe the chronic fatigue "elephant" based on the causes I've become most familiar with. Yet, I freely acknowledge that other causes are also important.

The Blind Men and the Elephant

It was six men of Indostan
To learning much inclined,
Who went to see the elephant
(Though all of them were blind),
That each by observation
Might satisfy his mind.

The first approached the elephant,
And happening to fall
Against his broad and sturdy side,
At once began to bawl:
"God bless me! but the elephant
Is nothing but a wall!"

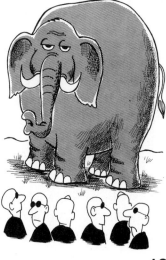

The second feeling of the tusk,
Cried: "Ho! What have we here
So very round and smooth and sharp?
To me 'tis mighty clear
This wonder of an elephant
Is very like a spear!"

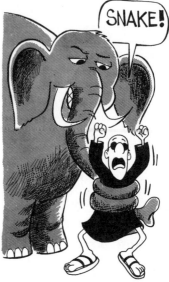

The third approached the animal,
And, happening to take
The squirming trunk within his
    hands,
Thus boldly up and spake:
"I see," quoth he, "the elephant
Is very like a snake!"

The fourth reached out his eager
    hand,
And felt about the knee:
"What most this wondrous beast is like
Is mighty plain," quoth he;
"'Tis clear enough, the elephant
Is very like a tree."

The fifth who chanced to touch the
    ear,
Said: "E'en the blindest man
Can tell what this resembles most;
Deny the fact who can
This marvel of an elephant
Is very like a fan!"

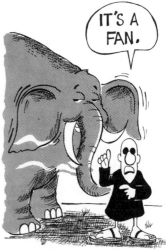

The sixth no sooner had begun
About the beast to grope,
Than, seizing on the swinging tail

That fell within his scope,
"I see," quoth he, "the
    elephant
Is very like a rope!"

And so these men of Indostan
Disputed loud and long.
Each of his own opinion
Exceeding stiff and strong,
Though each was partly in
    the right,
And all were in the wrong!

So, oft in theologic wars
The disputants, I ween,
Rant on in utter ignorance
Of what each other mean,
And prate about an elephant
Not one of them has seen!

John Godfrey Saxe

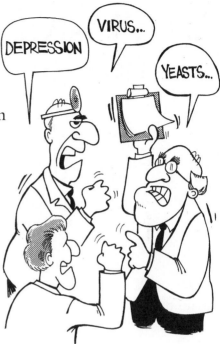

Don't Always Believe the "Experts"

If you review medical history, many discoveries made by observant people were often (even usually) greeted with skepticism, derision and hostility. As you may know, since chronic fatigue syndrome was first described in the 1980s, many skeptical physicians have said,

"People who complain of fatigue and aching in many parts of their body are not sick . . . there are no physical reasons to explain their symptoms." Here's a recent example of this sort of attitude.

In 1998 two "experts," Arthur J. Barsky, M.D., and Jonathan F. Borus, M.D., published a review entitled "Functional Somatic Syndromes" in the *Annals of Internal Medicine*.[1] They discussed what they called "poorly defined illnesses, such as chronic fatigue syndrome (CFS), fibromyalgia and the Gulf War syndrome." They stated that these illnesses are "self-diagnoses" and the suffering of these patients is little more than a "self-perpetuating, self-validating cycle" that is encouraged by sympathetic physicians.

David Bell, M.D., Vice-President of the American Association of Chronic Fatigue Syndrome (AACFS), and Charles Lapp, M.D., AACFS board member, responded. Here are excerpts which were published in an August/September 1999 issue of the AACFS newsletter and reprinted in the Winter 1999/2000 issue of the quarterly newsletter of the Wisconsin Chronic Fatigue Association, Inc.

"It should be obvious that the existence of an illness is not dependent upon knowledge of its etiology. Many illnesses, such as rheumatoid arthritis and multiple sclerosis are recognized, accepted and compassionately treated by physicians without a good understanding of the cause."

These physicians also pointed out that research has shown natural killer cells, cytokine abnormalities, MRI and SPECT abnormalities. They also noted that hypothalamic-pituitary-adrenal axis abnormalities are "emerging as an important area of new research." They also said that current textbooks "describe disabling fatigue associated with orthostatic intolerance, and a majority of CFS patients have postural tachycardia, postural hypotension, postural narrowing of the pulse pressure or decreased circulating blood volume."

In their continuing discussion they said, *"It is possible that CFS is a heterogeneous group of diseases"* (emphasis added). They also pointed out that even though there are laboratory abnormalities, a simple diagnostic test is not available.

Here are further excerpts.

"Clearly CFS is not straightforward depression, psychosis or panic disorder. . . The problem with the review by Drs. Barsky and Borus is that it magnifies . . . the distress of patients who are seeking adequate basic medical care . . . CFS and other somatic diseases are only beginning to be understood, and recognizing this illness in our patients should be a rewarding challenge.

"By making a diagnosis based on clinical presentation, doctors enable the patient to begin the process of coping. . . In summary, Barsky and Borus verbalized many prejudices felt by practicing physicians. But they voice only an opinion—an opinion that is unsupported by fact and substantially refuted by recent scientific data and clinical experience . . ."[2]

Two Examples from the 1700s and 1800s

Limes and Scurvy

In the 1740s, James Lind, a physician, learned by "serendipity" that putting limes and other fresh fruits and vegetables on British navy ships kept sailors from developing scurvy. Yet, the "experts" in the navy didn't believe him until 45 years later when they began putting limes on all British ships. Even then, the "experts" didn't know why limes worked and it wasn't until the 20th Century it was learned that they were a valuable source of vitamin C.

Childbed Fever

In the 1840s, a 26-year-old Austrian physician, Ignace Semelweiss, gave the medical students working under him the following instructions. *"Wash your hands carefully before you do a pelvic examination on women in labor."* Following these instructions, no more women on his obstetrical service died of "childbed fever." (This fatal disease was caused by the spread of streptococcal infections from the doctor's hands to the patients.)

On other obstetrical wards in the same hospital where these precautions were *not* taken, 10–20% of women in labor died. When Semelweiss told his chief (an "expert" in gynecology and obstetrics) about his observations, he was fired.

Examples During the 20th Century

Food and Chemical Sensitivities

In the 1940s Theron Randolph, a brilliant physician, noticed that food allergies played an important part in causing fatigue, irritability and other symptoms in adults and children under his care. He reported his findings in a number of publications, including the *Journal of Pediatrics*[3] and in a 1951 book, *Food Allergy.*[4]

In 1951, Randolph was fired from the allergy faculty of Northwestern University Medical School because the "expert" head of the faculty said that Randolph's teachings were " a pernicious influence on the medical students."

In 1961, Randolph published another book entitled *Human Ecology and Susceptibility to the Chemical Environment.*[5] In this book he carefully documented the role that environmental chemicals play in causing many chronic illnesses. In spite of this book, and many other articles and publications, the importance of his work was ignored by "experts" for over 30 years. But today, during the first decade of the 21st Century, professionals and nonprofessionals are recognizing the importance of Randolph's observations.

Vitamin B Complex in the Prevention of Heart Disease

In the 1960s, Kilmer McCully, M.D., described the role that elevated levels of homocysteine, a toxic product of protein metabolism, might play in causing premature death from heart disease in many people. He also noted that adequate amounts of vitamins B_6, B_{12} and folic acid could lower homocysteine levels and heart disease risk.

In discussing Dr. McCully's observations in the June 1999 issue of his monthly newsletter *Health and Healing,* Julian Whitaker, M.D., commented,

> "Thirty years ago, however, conventional medicine was so enmeshed in the cholesterol theory of heart disease that Dr. McCully's work was ignored—even ridiculed. When he refused to drop this 'trivial' area of research, he was eventually asked to leave Harvard. . . . In the past three years studies on homocysteine have been published in the most prestigious medical journals, and Dr. McCully's theory—and his recommendations

for supplemental B complex vitamins to protect against heart disease—is on the verge of being embraced by conventional medicine."[6]

More About Food Allergies and Sensitivities

In the 1960s and early 1970s, I published articles describing my observations on the relationship of food allergies to fatigue, irritability, headache and other symptoms in my patients. And in 1975, I published an article entitled "Food Allergy The Great Masquerader" in *Pediatric Clinics of North America*. Here are excerpts from that article.

> "In your office practice you'll see youngsters who . . . complain of headache, stomachache and aching in their legs and other muscles. You'll also see children whose parents bring them in for a check-up because their teacher may have complained, 'Johnny is so tired and sluggish, I wonder if he's getting enough rest?'"[7]

In the same issue of this publication Dr. Charles D. May of the University of Colorado, an expert allergist and immunologist, said,

> "Until we prove on scientific immunologic grounds that food is responsible for these reactions, rational physicians cannot accept them . . . Rather than calling food allergy the 'great masquerader' we should call it the current crutch for neurotic patients. And such has been the story of quackery and so it will always be until the last gaps in our knowledge are filled. We'll stamp it out in one area and it will crop up elsewhere. . . Energy and resources should be devoted to sound research undistracted by flimsy testimonials and preachers of dubious beliefs."[8]

At the annual meeting of the American Academy of Pediatrics in New York, November 8, 1977, the late Benjamin F. Feingold, M.D., in a presentation entitled "Hyperkinesis and Learning Disabilities Linked to the Ingestion of Artificial Foods and Flavors," described his own observations and reports by others which documented the relationship of dietary ingredients to nervous system symptoms in children.

Then, in the June/July 1978 issue of the *Journal of Learning Disabilities,* Doris J. Rapp, M.D., reported her experiences in an article entitled "Does Diet Affect Hyperactivity?" The article included her scientifically designed studies. In the concluding paragraph of the article she said,

> "Parents repeatedly volunteered that the ingestion of food coloring, sugar, and/or milk in particular, continue to be followed by hyperactivity."[9]

In my article in the May 1980 *Journal of Learning Disabilities* entitled "Can What a Child Eats Make Him Dull, Hyperactive or Stupid?" I published my observations on 182 children with behavior and learning problems who came to see me between January 1, 1973, and December 31, 1978.

> "Seventy percent (128) of the parents of children in the study reported that their child's hyperactivity was definitely related to dietary ingredients. The main causes were: sugar, colors, additives and flavors and milk. However many other foods were reported as causing trouble."[10]

In spite of my observations and those of Drs. Feingold and Rapp, most pediatricians and other physicians ignored or denied the relationship of food sensitivities to symptoms which bothered both children and adults.

Diet and ADHD

On through the 1980s and 1990s other "experts" continued to deny the relationship of sugar and other dietary factors to ADHD. Here's an example. In his 1996 book *Taking Charge of ADHD, The complete authoritative guide for parents,* Russell H. Barkley, Ph.D., University of Massachusetts Medical Center, discussed a number of "myths" under the heading "What Does Not Cause ADHD." Sugar was one of the myths he included.

In spite of the comments by Drs. May, Barkley and others, the role of food sensitivities and other dietary factors to health problems which affect countless children has been supported by many prestigious leaders. These include the late Frank Oski, M.D., Chairman of Pediatrics, Johns Hopkins; Walter W. Tunnessen, Jr., M.D., Vice-President of the American Board of Pediatrics; William "Ted" Kniker, M.D., University of Texas (San Antonio); Michael F. Jacobson, Ph.D., CSPI, Washington, DC; and, Joseph A. Bellanti, M.D., Professor of Pediatrics, Allergy and Immunology, Georgetown University Medical Center.

In the 1990s scientific studies were published that document the relationship of diet to nervous system symptoms in children. These include a report by Marvin Boris, M.D., and Francine S. Mandel, Ph.D., who found that 19 of 26 children with ADHD (73%) responded favorably to an elimination diet (p. 001). A double-blind, placebo-controlled food challenge was completed in 16 children.[11]

Another study reported in the *Journal of Pediatrics* by Katherine S. Rowe and Kenneth J. Rowe found that a 21-day, double-blind, placebo-controlled study showed that behavioral changes in irritability, restlessness and sleep disturbances were associated with the ingestion of tartrazine in some children.[12]

In 1993, C.M. Carter and colleagues published their observations on the relationship of diet to attention deficit disorder. Here's an excerpt from their conclusion.

"The results of a cross-over trial on 19 children showed a significant effect for the provoking foods to worsen ratings of behavior and to impair psychological test performance. This study shows that observations of change in behavior associated with diet made by parents . . . can be reproduced using double-blind methodology and objective assessments."[13]

Large Doses of Vitamin C

Over 30 years ago, the late Linus Pauling, Ph.D., the recipient of two Nobel Prizes, began to write and talk about the importance of larger doses of vitamin C. In a report in the January 1977 issue of *Executive Health,* "On Vitamin C and Cancer," he pointed out that a number of studies showed that large doses of vitamin C helped extend the life of patients with advanced cancer. He also said that these large doses of vitamin C could help people in the early stages of the disease.

In his article he referred to the observations of Dr. Ewan Cameron, a Scottish physician, who gave 100 patients with advanced cancer 10 grams of vitamin C a day. The patients who received these large doses *lived on an average four months longer than matched controls.*

During the 1970s and 1980s, Robert F. Cathcart, M.D., a California orthopedic surgeon, following Dr. Pauling's lead began using "mega" doses of vitamin C in individuals with suppressed immune systems. (Vitamin C: The nontoxic, antioxidant free radicals scavenger, *Medical Hypotheses,* 18:61–77, 1985)

In spite of these observations by Pauling, Cathcart and others, many "experts" today advise people to take no more than 60 mg. of vitamin C a day.

Yeast-Related Disorders

In a report entitled "Candidiasis Hypersensitivity Syndrome," approved by the Executive Committee of the American Academy of Allergy and Immunology (AAAI), a number of statements were made, including,

> "1. The concept is speculative and unproven. 2. The basic elements of the syndrome could apply to almost all sick patients at some time. 3. There's no published proof that *Candida albicans* is responsible for the syndrome."[14]

The American College of Allergy and Immunology published an identical proposed Position Statement and the Committee on Scientific Affairs of the American Medical Association published a similar negative opinion.

In response to these statements, I prepared a nine-page answer to their negative statements. In spite of my response, these organizations gave no indication that they would like additional information or would like to hear "the other side of the coin."

They have insisted on placebo-controlled, double-blind studies "proving" that *Candida albicans* is responsible for health problems which affect many people. Yet, there's considerable support for the importance of clinical trials—even unblinded trials. For example, in September 1978 the Office of Technology Assessment (OTA), Congress of the United States, in an article entitled "Assessing the Efficacy and Safety of Medical Technologies," stated,

> "It has been estimated that only 10–20% of all procedures currently used in medical practice have been shown to be efficacious by a controlled trial."

In an earlier report, OTA summarized the importance of informal methods of evaluation as follows:

> *". . . Personal experience is the primary method that determines whether or not a medical technology is adopted into widespread practice.* (emphasis added)
>
> ". . . Some procedures are so effective in restoring function that few would question their social utility.
>
> ". . . For a disease for which the natural history is fairly well known, and the benefits of a new technology are dramatic, alternative methods of evaluation (as compared to controlled trials) may be appropriate."[15]

Further support for clinical trials can be found in an editorial, "The Gold Standard," by Gene H. Stollerman, M.D., Professor of Medicine, Boston University. In his comments he said,

> "As the insights of medical bioscience and technology increase our medical powers, I find renewed strength in my medical skills. The medical history has become more focused and incisive as we learn better questions to ask . . . *Clinical experience is the 'gold standard' on which patient care should be based.*"[16]

Since the 1985 report by allergy "experts" was published, there have been a number of reports which support the relationship of superficial yeast infections to a number of chronic disorders. These include asthma, autism, chronic fatigue, endometriosis, fibromyalgia, headache, interstitial cystitis, multiple sclerosis and psoriasis.

A Final Comment

In an article, "The Tomato Effect," published in the Journal of the American Medical Association by James S. Goodwin, M.D., and Jean M. Goodwin, M.D., MPH, the authors stated,

> "The tomato effect in medicine occurs when an efficacious treatment for a certain disease is ignored or rejected because it does not 'make sense.'"

And they pointed out that pharmaceutical companies often recommend the use of a particular drug based on the results of laboratory studies rather than on its effectiveness in clinical trials. And they said,

"What gets lost in such discussions are the only three issues that matter in picking a therapy. Does it help? How toxic is it? How much does it cost? In this atmosphere we're at risk of rejecting a safe, inexpensive, effective therapy in favor of an alternative treatment, perhaps less efficacious and more toxic."[17]

See also the comments on nutritional supplements by Dr. James Goodwin and Tangum on pages 89–91.

REFERENCES

1. Barsky, A. J. and Borus, J. F., "Functional Somatic Syndromes," *Annals of Internal Medicine,* 1999; 130:910–921.

2. Bell, D. and Lapp, C., *Lifeline,* Quarterly newsletter of the Wisconsin Chronic Fatigue Syndrome Association, Inc., Vol. 12, No. 4, Winter 1999/2000, pp. 7–8. Office address: 1001 W. Main St., Suite B, Sun Prairie, WI 53590, Website: www.wicfs.me.org. E-mail: wicf.me@execpc.com.

3. Randolph, T. G., "Allergy as the Causative Factor of Fatigue, Irritability, and Behavior Problems in Children," 1947, *Journal of Pediatrics,* Vol. 32, pp. 560–572.

4. Rinkel, H. J., Randolph, T. G. and Zeller, M., *Food Allergy,* Charles C. Thomas, Springfield, IL., 1951.

5. Randolph, T., *Human Ecology and Susceptibility to the Chemical Environment,* Charles C. Thomas, Springfield, IL., 1961.

6. Whitaker, J., *Health & Healing,* June 1999.

7. Crook, W. G., "Food Allergy The Great Masquerader," *Pediatric Clinics of North America,* 22:219–226, 1975.

8. May, C., *Pediatric Clinics of North America,* February 1975.

9. Rapp, D., "Does Diet Affect Hyperactivity?" *Journal of Learning Disabilities,* June/July 1978.

10. Crook, W. G., "Can What A Child Eats Make Him Dull, Hyperactive or Stupid?," *Journal of Learning Disabilities,* May 1980.

11. Boris, M. and Mandel, F. S., "Foods and Additives Are Common Causes of the Attention Deficit/Hyperactivity Disorder in Children," *Annals of Allergy,* 1994; 72:462–468.

12. Rowe, K. S. and Rowe, K. J., "Synthetic Food Coloring and Behavior: A dose response effect in a double-blind, placebo-controlled, repeat measure study," *Journal of Pediatrics, 1994; 125:691–698.*

13. Carter, C. M., et al. "Effects of a few food diet in attention deficit disorder," *Archives of Diseases of Childhood,* 1993; 69:564–568.

14. The Practice Standards Committee, American Academy of Allergy and Immunology, "Candidiasis Hypersensitivity Syndrome," *J. Allergy Clin. Immunol.,* 1986;78:271–273.

15. "Assessing the Efficacy and Safety of Medical Technologies," Office of Technology Assessment (OTA), Congress of the United States, September, 1978.

16. Stollerman, G. H., "The Gold Standard," *Hospital Practice,* Vol. 20, No. 1A, January 30, 1985, page 9.

17. Goodwin, J. S., M.D. and Goodwin, J. M., M.D., MPH, "The Tomato Effect," *JAMA,* Vol. 251:18, pp. 2287–2290, May 11, 1984.

Chronic Fatigue and Food Sensitivities

left Johns Hopkins in 1949 and opened my pediatric office in Jackson, Tennessee. I saw children of all ages with many different types of problems. Although I was able to help many of these children, there were others who puzzled me—children I failed to help. One such youngster (I'll call him Tom) came to see me four or five times during 1955. His complaints included fatigue, weakness and inability to get out of bed in the morning. He also complained of headache, irritability, abdominal pain and muscle aches.

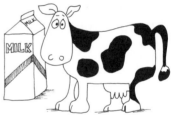

I went over Tom with a fine tooth comb and put him through a battery of laboratory tests. When all proved to be negative, Tom's mother, Aileen, said, "I think that drinking a lot of cow's milk is contributing to Tom's fatigue, headache and other symptoms."

Although I didn't understand how or why milk could cause Tom's problems, I agreed that experimenting with his diet made sense.

A week later, Aileen called and said, "Tom is like a different child. He bounced out of bed this morning whistling. No headache, muscle aches or belly aches." I was astounded because I learned that sensitivities to common foods could provoke fatigue and other symptoms.

Not long after that, as I thumbed through the November 1954 issue of *Pediatric Clinics of North America,* I came across an article by a University of Kansas physician, Frederic Speer, entitled "The Allergic Tension-Fatigue Syndrome." In his article, Dr. Speer described several patients with fatigue, irritability and other symptoms who improved dramatically when common foods were eliminated from their diet.[1]

Much to my surprise, I found 21 references at the end of Speer's article. Among the reports he cited was an article by Albert Rowe, Sr., of Oakland, California, who in 1930 described his experiences in studying and treating patients with fatigue, headache, depression, abdominal pain, diarrhea, intestinal gas, nasal congestion, wheezing, and other symptoms.[2]

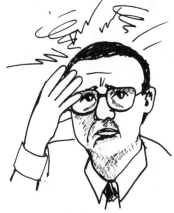

Rowe reported that many of these patients improved—often dramatically—when they avoided wheat, corn, milk, egg and other common foods. Rowe called this disorder "allergic toxemia." And he continued to write and talk about food-related fatigue until his death in the early 1970s.

Following in Rowe's footsteps, Herbert Rinkel[3] and Theron Randolph[4,5] in the 1940s described patients with food-related fatigue, depression and other symptoms which could be relieved using 5-to-10-day elimination diets.

As I read and reread the Speer article and the reports of other physicians who described food-related fatigue and other symptoms, I was amazed. And I said to myself, "I wonder if a food sensitivity could be responsible for Marlene's drowsiness and fatigue . . . fatigue that makes her unable to sit at her desk at school, even though she's somehow able to keep up with her work. Or George's lethargy, which keeps him from going out and playing with the rest of the gang."

So I began putting a number of my tired, dreamy, irritable, inattentive patients on one-week trial diets. Although I didn't help all of them, I was excited because I began to receive reports from mothers who said, "Susie's like a different child. But when I give her chocolate milk, corn chips, wheat, or eggs, her symptoms return."

I collected and summarized my findings on 23 of these patients and presented them at the Allergy Section of the American Academy of Pediatrics in October 1958, and I published my findings on 50 of these tired, irritable children in *Pediatrics* in 1961.[6]

+ A diagnosis of food sensitivity was made in the following manner. Symptoms and signs were relieved by eliminating suspected foods from the diet for 5 to 12 days and then reproduced by returning the foods to the child, one each day the following week.

During the 1960s and 1970s, I saw and helped hundreds of my patients using carefully designed and properly executed elimination diets. I reported my observations in *Pediatric Annals* and the *Pediatric Clinics of North America*.[7,8] Moreover, I found that food sensitivities could affect just about any and every part of the body. *Common symptoms included fatigue, drowsiness and depression in some youngsters and irritability, short attention span and overactivity in others*. And in some patients, these symptoms would alternate.

During the 1960s, 1970s and 1980s, a number of physicians in practice and in academic centers described their findings on children with food-induced fatigue and other symptoms. Included among the academicians were William C. Deamer,[9a,b,] professor of pediatrics, University of California, San Francisco; John W. Gerrard,[10] professor of pediatrics, University of Saskatchewan; Douglas Sandberg,[11] professor of pediatrics, University of Miami; Frank A. Oski and Walter Tunnessen, Jr., professors of pediatrics at the Upstate Medical Center of New York, Syracuse.

Dr. Deamer, a pediatric allergist, became interested in the Allergic Tension-Fatigue Syndrome in the early 1960s. In the next two decades he presented his observations in scientific exhibits and in articles and commentaries in the medical literature. In discussing recurrent abdominal pain, headache and limb pains he said,

> "In one series of 96 children with the Allergic Tension-Fatigue Syndrome seen in our Pediatric Allergy Clinic and privately, the six most common complaints—other than respiratory tract symptoms—were, in order: headache, 61%; recurrent abdominal pain, 58%; pallor, 52%; fatigue or tiredness, 47%; limb pains, 36%. . .
>
> "All 96 patients were successfully treated for the stated symptoms by elimination of specific food allergens . . . . milk and chocolate in particular. In most instances, either a sibling or a parent had a history of similar symptoms attributable to food sensitivity."[9b]

In 1977, Frank A. Oski, M.D., who was at that time chairman of the department of pediatrics at the Upstate Medical Center at Syracuse, expressed concern over what he felt to be the excessive emphasis on milk in the diet of American children. He summarized his thoughts in a book entitled *Don't Drink Your Milk*.[12] In his book, Dr. Oski cited reports that showed that milk caused health problems for a variety of reasons, including excessive fat and lactose intolerance.

He also reviewed and cited my article "Food Allergy, The Great Masquerader," which was published in the *Pediatric Clinics of North America* in February 1975. In a chapter of his book entitled "Milk and the Tension-Fatigue Syndrome" Dr. Oski commented,

> "Most people, including physicians, believe that allergies to food . . . produce only classical symptoms as skin rashes, respiratory symptoms, or gastrointestinal disorders. There is a growing body of evidence, however, to suggest that certain allergies may manifest themselves primarily as changes in personality, emotions, or in one's general sense of well-being. . . .
>
> *"The child or adult with motor fatigue always seems to feel weak and tired. The child may interrupt his playing in order to rest or may even have to put his head down on the desk at school because he's feeling so tired. Excessive drowsiness and torpor are typical. These children are particularly listless in the morning. They're difficult to awaken and appear never to have a good night's sleep.* . . .[emphasis added]
>
> "Although the Tension-Fatigue Syndrome is the most common manifestation of food allergy, it is by no means the only one. Vague, recurrent abdominal pains, repeated headaches, aching muscles and joints and even bedwetting have been observed as symptoms of food allergy."

One of Dr. Oski's colleagues at Syracuse and later at Johns Hopkins, Walter W. Tunnessen, Jr., found that he could help his own child and other tired, polysymptomatic patients by identifying foods that were triggering their symptoms and removing them from the diet. And in an article in *CLINI-PEARLS,* in presenting the history of an eight-year-old boy with lethargy and fatigue to a group of young pediatricians, Dr. Tunnessen made the following comments.

> "An eight-year-old boy is brought to your office by both of his parents. For the previous six months they have noted increased lethargy and decreasing energy and tolerance to exercise. A number of other physicians have been consulted, but nothing concrete has been found. The parents are concerned

that the child has a serious underlying disorder and implore you to examine him thoroughly. . . .

"On examination, the child . . . sits quietly on the examining table and looks tired and pale. Dark circles rim his eyelids. Except for some shotty cervical adenopathy, the results of the physical examination are completely normal. . . . (Laboratory tests are also normal.)

"Whenever both parents accompany a child to the office, I know the index of parental concern has reached titanic proportions. The father extols his son's past performance in a recreational wrestling program. Now the boy is barely able to wrestle five minutes before becoming exhausted. The mother pipes in that *he rarely joins other children in after-school play. . . .*" [emphasis added]

"Where do we go from here? Maybe the problem does have an emotional basis, but before we label this child as such, consider the great masquerader, food allergy. . . . I cannot prove it with esoteric or even routine laboratory tests . . . the proof of the pudding . . . is in some simple dietary elimination . . . a benign procedure, most often painless and not requiring hospitalization and downright inexpensive.

"*The culprits I find most common are milk, chocolate and eggs, although cane sugar, corn and wheat should also be considered. Removing these foods from the diet a few at a time for a week or two is all that is necessary. Should the child improve—the eliminated foods are reintroduced . . . Relief of symptoms further supports the diagnosis.* [emphasis added]

"I, too, had been a doubting Thomas until my son responded to dietary elimination . . . The boy presented in the case above was taken off milk, chocolate and eggs. Within a week he was a new person."[13]

Like many pediatricians interested in allergy, in the 1970s I began to see more adult patients. These included not only men and women with hay fever, asthma and skin rashes, but also people with a variety of other complaints, including fatigue, headache, muscle aches and depression. I was delighted and excited when many of these patients improved when they eliminated common foods from their diets.

I was also able to help many tired, polysymptomatic adult patients by teaching them how to avoid tobacco smoke, insecticides and odorous chemicals. Others I helped by recommending lifestyle changes, nutritional supplements and using allergy extracts and vaccines. But I didn't help every person who came to see me, as you'll see in the following chapter, "The Yeast Connection to Chronic Fatigue."

REFERENCES

1. Speer, F., "The Allergic Tension-Fatigue Syndrome," *Pediatric Clinics of North America,* 1:1029, 1954.

2. Rowe, A.H., Sr., "Allergic Toxemia and Migraine Due to Food Allergy," *California and Western Medicine,* 33:785, 1930.

3. Rinkel, H.J., "Food Allergy: The role of food allergy in internal medicine," *Annals of Allergy,* 2:115, 1944.

4. Randolph, T.G., "Fatigue and Weakness of Allergic Origin (Allergic toxemia)," *Annals of Allergy,* 3:418, 1945.

5. Randolph, T.G., "Allergies as the Causative Factor of Fatigue, Irritability and Behavior Problems in Children," *Journal of Pediatrics,* 32:266, 1948.

6. Crook, W.G., et al., "Systemic Manifestations Due to Allergy: Report of fifty patients and a review of the literature on the subject (allergic toxemia and the allergic tension-fatigue syndrome)," *Pediatrics,* 27:790–799, 1961.

7. Crook, W.G., "The Allergic Tension-Fatigue Syndrome," *Pediatric Annals,* October 1974.

8. Crook, W.G., "Food Allergy: The Great Masquerader," *Pediatric Clinics of North America,* 22:22–27, 1975.

9a. Deamer, W.C., "Pediatric Allergy: Some Impressions Gained Over a 37-Year Period," *Pediatrics* 48:930–938, 1971.

9b. Deamer, W.C. *Pediatrics,* 52:307, 1973. (Letters)

10. Gerrard, J.W., *Understanding Allergies,* Springfield, IL, Charles C. Thomas, pp. 14–17, 1973.

11. Sandberg, D.H., "Recurrent Abdominal Pain: The current controversy," (Letters), *Pediatrics,* 51:307, 1973.

12. Oski, F.A., *Don't Drink Your Milk,* Molica Press, Ltd., 1914 Teall Ave., Syracuse, NY 13203, pp. 85–88, 1977, 1983.

13. Tunnessen, W.W., "An Eight-Year-Old Boy with Lethargy and Fatigue, *CliniPearls,* Vol. 2, No. 8, July/August, 1979.

The Yeast Connection to Chronic Fatigue

In 1976, a 35-year-old woman (I'll call her Linda Jones) came to my office seeking help. In fact, she was "sick all over." Although she showed some improvement when she changed her diet and cleaned up the chemical pollutants in her home, she continued to experience symptoms of many sorts, including devastating fatigue.

Because of her continuing problem, she moved away and I lost contact with her. Then in the fall of 1979, I learned from one of her former neighbors that she had moved back to West Tennessee and that she was healthy, active and energetic. So I called her up and said, "Ms. Jones, I hear you're doing well. I'd love to know what you did to get your life and health back on track." And she replied, "I'll tell you, Dr. Crook, and I won't even charge you for an office visit!"

When Ms. Jones came to my office she handed me a copy of an article published in a little known Canadian medical journal.[1] It was written by C. Orian Truss, M.D., a Birmingham, Alabama, specialist in internal medicine.* She said, "Dr. Crook, read this paper. It contains information which will enable you to help some of your difficult, tired, irritable and depressed patients."

Dr. Truss' report told how the common yeast *Candida albicans,* growing on the warm interior membranes of the body

---

*See also Sections III and VII.

(especially the gut and the vagina), could play an important role in causing problems in many parts of the body. Symptoms in patients with candida-related health problems included fatigue, PMS, depression and disorders of the immune, endocrine and nervous systems.

After reading the paper, I called Dr. Truss to obtain additional information. And I asked, "How do you make a diagnosis of a candida-related health problem? Are there tests that help?" In responding, Dr. Truss said in effect,

> "Since everyone has some yeast in the digestive tract, and most women have it in the vagina, smears and cultures do not help significantly in making the diagnosis. Instead it's suspected in any person who has received repeated courses of broad spectrum antibiotic drugs, such as the tetracyclines, ampicillin, amoxicillin, Keflex or Ceclor. Birth control pills and steroids also encourage the growth of candida.
>
> *"It is further suspected in the person with such a medical history who develops fatigue, headache, depression and other symptoms who has failed to respond to multiple diagnostic evaluations and therapies. Finally, it is confirmed by the response of such patients to a special diet and the oral antifungal medication nystatin."*

I was skeptical about some of the things Dr. Truss told me. Yet, because I had many patients who seemed to fit the category he described, I was interested. So I began to place a number of my tired, polysymptomatic patients on the treatment program recommended by Dr. Truss. Within about six months I had successfully treated 20 such patients and I was delighted and astounded at their response.

Because of the response of these patients I began to treat—and help—other patients (especially women between 25 and 45) who complained of fatigue, muscle aches, poor memory, mental

confusion, depression, headache, digestive disorders, sexual dysfunction and other symptoms which made them feel "sick all
over." My treatment program in working with these patients
featured a sugar-free special diet and nystatin.

During the early 1980s, Truss' observations spread to other
physicians in the United States, England, Australia and New
Zealand. And hundreds of them found that a special diet and
the antifungal medications nystatin and Nizoral (ketoconazole)
helped their patients

My ability to help these patients and the interest of dozens of
physicians and their patients led me to write *The Yeast Connection*
(published in hardback in 1983 and 1985, and in paperback in
1986). During the mid and late 1980s, many people who had
read this book wrote to me and said, "Dr. Crook, we've read
that the Epstein-Barr virus (EBV) and other viruses may cause
people to develop an illness similar to those described in your
book."

To get an additional opinion on the relationship of candida
yeasts to viral infections, I consulted Elmer Cranton, M.D., a
graduate of Harvard Medical School and editor (at that time)
of the *Journal of Advancement in Medicine*. In responding, he
said in effect,

> "In treating patients in my practice with yeast-related ill-
> ness, I find that close to one-fourth had viral infections. *There
> is also no question that the health problems of the vast majority of
> these patients are primarily candida related. I feel that the chronic
> yeast condition weakens the immunity and causes latent viruses to
> become activated* . . .
>
> "I'm not certain which comes first, the chicken or the egg.
> That is, did the virus lower immunity and cause a person to
> become susceptible to yeast or vice versa? I'm sure that it must
> occur in both directions."

At a CFS conference in San Francisco on April 15, 1989, Carol Jessop, M.D., told of her experiences in treating 1100 patients with CFS. All of these patients met the Centers for Disease Control diagnostic criteria for CFS.

In reviewing the histories of the patients, she found that 80% took recurrent courses of antibiotics during childhood. She also said that irritable bowel syndrome, vaginal yeast infections, headache and the premenstrual syndrome were extremely common.

Jessop treated her patients with a special diet (no alcohol, sugar, fruit or fruit juice). They were also given 200 mg of ketoconazole (Nizoral) once daily. Eighty-four percent of the patients showed a greater than 70% improvement. The average length of therapy was five months.

In her concluding remarks, Dr. Jessop stated,

> "CFS may represent a multitude of symptoms which are manifested with the presence of a toxin released by *Candida albicans*."

In the Foreword to my 1992 book *Chronic Fatigue Syndrome and the Yeast Connection*, Jessop said,

> "This book does not claim that the yeast *Candida albicans* is *the* cause of CFS, however, it does explain the role of multiple entities, yeast overgrowth, intestinal parasites, unchecked viral infections, food allergies and chemical sensitivities and how they can result in the immune dysregulation we refer to as CFS."

My Comments: *I realize that antifungal medication does not provide a "quick fix" for every person with fatigue, muscle aches, poor memory and other symptoms. Yet, based on my own experiences in practice, and those of C. Orian Truss, Elmer Cranton, Jacob Teitel-*

baum and other physicians, I'm certain that a comprehensive treatment program which features a special diet and antifungal medication will help many people who are sick and tired, including those who have been labeled "chronic fatigue syndrome."

REFERENCE

1. Truss, C.O. "Tissue Injury Induced by *Candida albicans:* Mental and Neurologic Manifestations." *Journal of Orthomolecular Psychiatry,* 7:17 37, 1978

Women and Chronic Fatigue

Without exception researchers and practicing physicians have found that recurrent or persistent fatigue affects women more often than men. And women between the ages of 25 and 50 seem especially apt to complain of being tired. Why is there such a gender difference? *Candida albicans* may provide a part of the answer.

✦ Hormonal changes associated with the normal menstrual cycle encourage yeast colonization.

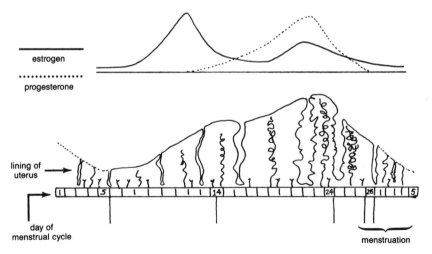

✦ Birth control pills and pregnancy promote yeast overgrowth.
✦ Yeasts thrive on the warm interior membranes of the body, including the vagina.
✦ The anatomy of the female urinary tract makes women

much more apt to develop urinary infections. Antibiotics (which promote yeast growth) are usually used in treating such infections.

✦ Women are more likely to establish a relationship with a physician. This may make them more apt to receive antibiotic drugs for respiratory infections.

Vaginal Yeast Infections and Chronic Fatigue

According to recent reports in the press and advertisements on TV and in women's magazines, 22 million American women are affected by recurrent vaginal yeast infections. Moreover, the incidence of these infections appears to be increasing.

The number of people with chronic fatigue—especially young women—is also increasing. Here's a possible connection.

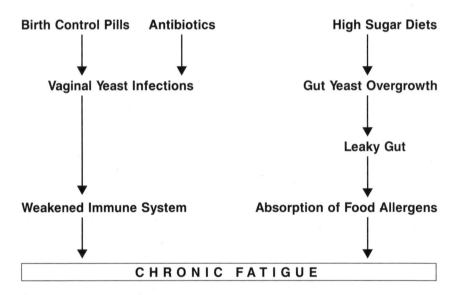

The South Carolina Report

In a three-page clinical report in the *Journal of the South Carolina Medical Association*, Martin H. Zwerling, M.D.,

Kenneth M. Owens, M.D. and Nancy H. Ruth, R.N., B.S., described their experiences in treating 79 private patients with yeast-related health problems. There were 53 women and 26 men, and all were patients from the private practice of the authors. Seventy of these patients had good to excellent results. Four dropped out of the study and were lost to followup, and five showed no improvement.

In introducing their report, these authors emphasized yeast-connected health problems in women, and stated,

> "Consider the following 'incurable' patient who has been treated by several specialists. A gynecologist is treating her recurrent vaginitis and irregular menstrual periods while an otolaryngologist is trying to control her external otitis and chronic rhinitis.
>
> "At the same time an internist is unsuccessfully attempting to manage symptoms of bloating, indigestion and abdominal pain and a dermatologist is struggling with bizarre skin rashes, hives and psoriasis.
>
> "Lastly, her psychiatrist has been unable to convince the patient that her 'nerves' are the cause of her extreme irritability, inability to concentrate and depression.
>
> "We have all been guilty of labeling such patients as 'psychosomatic' and since 'there is nothing physically wrong' conclude we can not cure them. Incurable? Not if you THINK YEAST. This patient and thousands like her are suffering from chronic candidiasis."

In discussing yeast-related problems, the authors stated,

> "Normally the yeast lives in quiet balance with its human host and the usual bacteria inhabiting the mucosal skin and G.I. tracts and cause no symptoms or apparent harm. However, when this delicate balance is disturbed, the yeasts are free to . . . release their toxins into the blood stream.

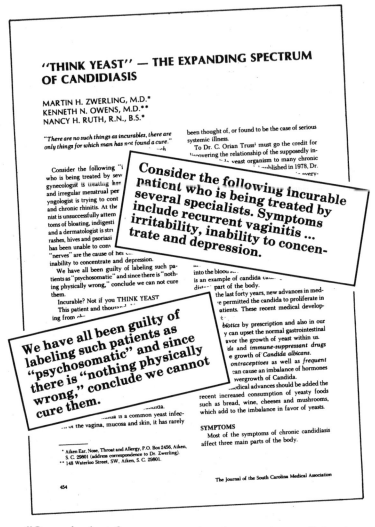

"THINK YEAST" — THE EXPANDING SPECTRUM OF CANDIDIASIS

MARTIN H. ZWERLING, M.D.*
KENNETH N. OWENS, M.D.**
NANCY H. RUTH, R.N., B.S.*

"There are no such things as incurables, there are only things for which man has not found a cure."

been thought of, or found to be the case of serious systemic illness.

To Dr. C. Orian Truss[1] must go the credit for discovering the relationship of the supposedly in-nocuous yeast organism to many chronic ... ...hlished in 1978, Dr.

Consider the following "i who is being treated by sev gynecologist is treating her and irregular menstrual per yngologist is trying to cont and chronic rhinitis. At the nist is unsuccessfully attem toms of bloating, indigesti and a dermatologist is str rashes, hives and psoriasi has been unable to con "nerves" are the cause of her inability to concentrate and depression.

> **Consider the following incurable patient who is being treated by several specialists. Symptoms include recurrent vaginitis ... irritability, inability to concentrate and depression.**

We have all been guilty of labeling such patients as "psychosomatic" and since there is "nothing physically wrong," conclude we can not cure them.

Incurable? Not if you THINK YEAST

This patient and thous... ing from ...

into the bloou... is an example of candida ca... dist... part of the body.

the last forty years, new advances in med-'e permitted the candida to proliferate in atients. These recent medical develop-

f...

biotics by prescription and also in our y can upset the normal gastrointestinal avor the growth of yeast within us. ds and *immune-suppressant* drugs e growth of *Candida albicans*. *ontraceptives* as well as *frequent* can cause an imbalance of hormones wergrowth of Candida. ...edical advances should be added the recent increased consumption of yeasty foods such as bread, wine, cheeses and mushrooms, which add to the imbalance in favor of yeasts.

> **We have all been guilty of labeling such patients as "psychosomatic" and since there is "nothing physically wrong," conclude we cannot cure them.**

...aida.

... is a common yeast infec-... on the vagina, mucosa and skin, it has rarely

SYMPTOMS

Most of the symptoms of chronic candidiasis affect three main parts of the body.

* Aiken Ear, Nose, Throat and Allergy, P.O. Box 2456, Aiken, S. C. 29801 (address correspondence to Dr. Zwerling).
** 148 Waterloo Street, SW, Aiken, S. C. 29801.

The Journal of the South Carolina Medical Association

454

"Over the last forty years new advances in medicine have permitted the candida to proliferate in certain patients. These recent developments are:

"1. *Antibiotics* by prescription and also in our food supply can upset the normal gastrointestinal flora and favor the growth of yeast within us.

"2. *Steroids* and *immune-suppressant* drugs stimulate the growth of *Candida albicans*.

"3. *Oral contraceptives,* as well as frequent pregnancies, can cause an imbalance of hormones which favor overgrowth of candida."[1]

The Michigan State University Study

While vaginal suppositories may relieve the symptoms of vaginitis, in many women the problem returns. And a study carried out at Michigan State University on 98 young women who complained of recurrent vaginitis appears to provide an explanation.

Here's an abstract of the Michigan State study published in the *Journal of the American Medical Association.*

159

Recurrent Vaginal Candidiasis

Importance of an Intestinal Reservoir

Mary Ryan Miles, MD; Linda Olsen, MS; Alvin Rogers, PhD

● To test the hypothesis that all cases of vaginal candidiasis ated with a "reservoir" of this organism in the bowel, feces and vaginal material were cultured for neously. Ninety-eight young women who were selected in sequence. The results a tured from the vagina, it was always found not isolated from the stool, it was never fou presented as an explanation for the recurre and thus a cure of vaginitis would not be pos of *C albicans* from the gut. The gut-reservoir c forms of candidiasis.

(*JAMA* 238:1836-1837, 1977)

Extending the gut reservoir concept, may explain other forms of candidiasis and the immunological phenomena found in some people.

CANDIDA ALBICANS is found so frequer ‚at its presence health in th as t ing th v

When *C. albicans* was cultured from the vagina it was always found in the stool.

This pap ‚e evidence that the intestin. acts as a reservoir for *C albicans*, where it may live in harmony with the rest of the host's fecal flora. Minor alterations in the milieu ‚f the host (ie, pregnancy and inges-‚re from commensal to ‚cutaneous sur-‚tes of in- ‚a, ie, per or results at vagi- ‚ur natu- ‚tant pres- ‚ the large is not likely remains the

...n was used for ... *C albicans.* This me- ‚signated to inhibit the growth ...ost micro-organisms but to allow the growth of *Candida* species. Yeast growth is evident as early as 24 hours after inocu-lation, but optimal growth may be ex-pected between five and seven days when incubated at 24 C. Approximately 1 gm of fecal material and swabs containing vagi-nal specimens were inoculated directly into the media. Chlamydospore formation on commeal plus polysorbate-80 agar was used for positive identification of *C albi-cans.*

RESULTS

Ninety-eight patients were in-volved in the study. Fifty-one (52%) were found to harbor *C albicans* in both vagina and fecal material; 46 (47%) were *Candida* free in both sites (Table 1). Thus, there was 100% corre-lation between the presence or ab-sence of *C albicans* in the feces and vagina of this population (Table 2).

A review of the patient's clinical records supported the recurrent na-ture of candidiasis. In approximately one third of the patients, there had been no prior laboratory confirmation

Vagin...

become one o... forms of vaginitis be... quently a recurrent problem sons that some persons present ... repeated episodes of vaginitis and other forms of mucocutaneous candi-diasis are not known although precip-itating events are known. Cellular and humoral immunological data are rapidly accumulating,'' but as yet, ‚ributed little knowledge in ‚anesis or

bowe... as long as only treatment ta...

PATIENTS AND METHODS

Patients.—Healthy, nonpregnant, female patients, 18 to 20 years of age, who pre-

‚ Incidence of C Albicans Isolation From Stool and Vagina

	Vagina No. (%)

"To test the hypothesis that all cases of vaginal candidiasis are associated with a 'reservoir' of this organism in the bowel, paired specimens of feces and vaginal material were cultured for *Candida albicans* simultaneously. Ninety-eight young women who complained of recurrent vaginitis were selected in sequence. The results showed that if *C. albicans* was cultured from the vagina, it was always found in the stool.

"Conversely, if it was not isolated from the stool, it was never found in the vagina. These data are presented as an explanation for the recurrent nature of *candida* vaginitis. And thus a cure for vaginitis would not be possible without prior eradication of *C. albicans* from the gut. The gut reservoir concept may well apply to other forms of candidiasis."

In their concluding comments, the authors of this article stated,

"Of economic importance is the knowledge that candida vaginitis cannot be cured by vigorously treating the vagina. Millions of consumer dollars are spent yearly in vain in hope of accomplishing this. . . . *Extending the gut reservoir concept may explain other forms of candidiasis and the immunological phenomena found in some people.*"[2] [emphasis added]

The Yeast Connection to PMS

In the mid 1980s, Jay Schinfeld, M.D., who at that time was a member of the faculty at the University of Tennessee Health Science Center, began a study on patients in the university's PMS clinic. He published his observations in July 1987 and presented them at the Candida Update Conference in Memphis in September 1988. *Symptoms in Dr. Schinfeld's patients included fatigue, depression, migraine, anxiety, loss of libido, mood swings, bloating and food cravings.* Here's a summary of Dr. Schinfeld's observations.

"We performed a study at the University of Tennessee in which 32 women with severe premenstrual syndrome and a history of vaginal candidiasis for whom prior standardized therapy had failed were treated with oral anti-candida agents and yeast elimination diets.

"Treated patients showed significant physical and psychological improvement over untreated controls... Further anecdotal reports have suggested that treatment of chronic candidiasis has resulted in prompt cessation of infertility."[3]

REFERENCES

1. Zwerling, M.H., Owens, K.N. and Ruth, N.H., "Think Yeast"—The Expanding Spectrum of Candidiasis, *J. South Carolina Med. Association,* pp. 454–456, 1984.

2. Miles, M.R., Olsen, L. and Rogers, A., "Recurrent Vaginal Candidiasis: Importance of an Intestinal Reservoir," *JAMA,* 238:1836–1837, October 28, 1977.

3. Schinfeld, J., "Possible Links of Chronic Candidiasis to PMS and Infertility," *The Female Patient,* pp. 66–73, July 1987.

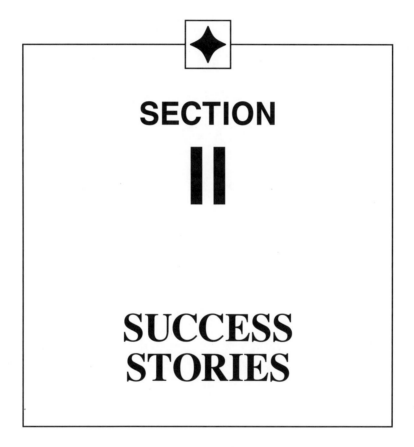

SECTION

II

SUCCESS STORIES

Personal Triumphs

MARGARET

"May of 1989 was the beginning of two years that I will never forget. During the previous year, I had been treated with various antibiotics which led to a continuous yeast infection.

"My headaches were so severe I used an ice bag to try to get relief. My muscles were so tender I could not stand to be touched. Life was miserable and I started to search for answers and for help.

"My condition continued to worsen until I could not talk on the phone for more than five minutes. Just walking outside took major effort. When I went to the store I had to go in a wheelchair. I could not do my housework or even cook, much less grocery shop. I had severe spells of being unable to breathe, feeling as each breath would be my last.

"The fatigue was sometimes so severe that I could not get out of bed no matter how bad I wanted to. Before this came on me I was a very happy woman who loved taking care of my home, babysitting my granddaughter, and being involved in my church.

"My personal physician was kind and caring and did a series of tests, but with nothing showing positive. He finally diagnosed me with chronic fatigue syndrome, which was just getting its name at the time. In an effort to help, he gave me a prescription for Prozac. I chose not to have it filled. I have a strong faith in God and had many people praying for me. I never lost faith that the answers were out there.

"Then, through a series of events, I was led by a friend to purchase your book *The Yeast Connection*. This information was as if it had been written about me. After reading, marking and highlighting many pages, I went back to my doctor and asked for nystatin. He refused because of the possible side effects.

"Convinced that this was my answer, and with my doctor's approval, I followed the sugar-free diet to the letter. I would not even eat ketchup because it had corn syrup in it. For a whole year I ate nothing sweet.

"I was also helped by a yeast-control product from a health food store which contained caprylic acid, garlic and other ingredients. I continued to follow the recommendations in your book and started to improve. With the help of another doctor I learned that I was allergic to yeasts, dairy, and especially to egg white. This was a tremendous revelation and explanation to my previously described symptoms. Prior to a series of antibiotics and yeast infections, I had no food sensitivities. So my life 'turned around' . . . *the diet was the most important part of my treatment program.*

"Today, October 2000, I continue to watch my diet, avoid chemicals and food additives and foods I'm allergic to. I also continue supplements everyday which have helped me very much in maintaining my well being and energy. I now babysit five-year-old twin grandchildren, their 18-month-old little brother and their two-year-old cousin. Also, my 89-year-old mother still lives with me as well.

"I work with 12 teenagers in our church and serve as the director of a very active Puppet Team. I am also chairman of our community National Day of Prayer every May. Last, but not least, I am now a member of the Advisory Board of Dr. Crook's International Health Foundation."

JOYCE

In August 1992 this 35-year-old woman called me and said, "I've had severe myasthenia gravis for over twenty years." Her symptoms included complete nasal voice with no control of her facial muscles.

She was also troubled by double vision, migraine headaches and stomach aches. During the years following her diagnosis she developed other problems, including recurrent yeast infections, constipation, depression and severe body weakness.

In spite of many therapies, including daily prednisone and gamma globulin by intravenous drip once a week, Joyce continued to be troubled by many symptoms including PMS, headache, irritability, panic attacks, poor memory and indescribable body weakness and fatigue.

"I had to be vertical most of the day. I could not carry on normal duties, including cooking and cleaning. Some days I had to stay in bed all day; folding a load of clothes required too much energy. I had to quit my job."

Early in 1993, Joyce saw Dr. C. Orian Truss in Birmingham. Following a careful history and examination, he prescribed nystatin and a restricted diet. Within a short time she reported 100% more energy and no more weak days. In March 1993 she went on a ski vacation and skied from 7:30 in the morning until 4:30 in the afternoon. By contrast, seven months earlier she couldn't sit up or do other normal household duties.

I've followed Joyce by phone over the years and although she's had a few ups and downs, her progress has been remarkable. In October 2000, she said, "I'm doing great! I still must take huge doses of nystatin and follow my diet. I'm eager to share my story with others, as I feel it will give them hope and help."

GEORGE

"In my teen years I took tetracycline for two years because of acne. Then in my early 20s I developed headache, fatigue, abdominal pain and bloating. I just didn't feel good. Some days

I'd almost fall asleep on my desk at work and I was too tired to exercise.

"Check ups by my family doctor and a gastroenterologist, who carried out an endoscopic examination, showed no abnormalities. So I began feeling like a hypochondriac. I felt that a 28-year-old with a darn good job and a beautiful girlfriend should feel a lot better than I did. But I didn't know where to turn.

"Then my sister said, 'George because of all those antibiotics, your health problems are probably yeast-related.' So I picked up *The Yeast Connection Handbook* at a health food store and I was impressed. I eliminated sugar and made other dietary changes. I also started taking caprylic acid, probiotics, vitamins and minerals and flax seed oil.

"Thank you so much for your help. My health and my life are much, much better."

PAULA

This 38-year-old Nashville, Tennessee, business woman worked ten hours a day, ran 15 miles a week and enjoyed an active, personal and professional life. In her late 20s, after taking tetracycline for acne for 18 months, Paula developed concentration problems, anxiety and fatigue. *Her symptoms were disabling and she had to give up her job and stay in bed most of every day for a year.*

Through networking she obtained my home address and told me her story and asked for help. I gave her the name of an empathetic physician who prescribed nystatin, a sugar-free special diet and nutritional supplements. Within a short time, Paula began to improve and within a few months she was back at work.

Here are excerpts from a letter Paula sent me in 1997. "Thank you and the International Health Foundation for putting me in touch with the physician who helped me. Rather than feeling like a limp washcloth, I'm now back to 95% of where I started from. Enclosed with my letter is a small check for you to give to the International Health Foundation. I strongly believe in your efforts so you can count on me as an annual contributor."

During a phone visit in October 2000, Paula said, "I'm working full time in a very responsible job. Although I had a slight setback after taking an antibiotic, I'm now back on track, traveling and fulfilling many job responsibilities. Thanks again for your help. Without it I do not know where I would be today."

ALBERTA

"I was the typical CFS profile. An educated female in her 30s and a workaholic. I graduated from law school and was a major in the U.S. Army. Although I never took sick leave, the doctors often gave me antibiotics for repeated urinary tract infections. I then became desperately ill. I slept 14 hours a day and my head felt as though it would burst. I ached all over, especially in my joints. _Just getting dressed exhausted me._

"Although I suffered from many different symptoms, including fatigue, headache, nasal congestion and much, much more, the doctors who checked me over would always say, 'Nothing's wrong.' I felt so bad I even considered suicide. I didn't know how I would ever be able to perform my job, but I had to work to support myself.

"Then I began reading everything I could. And I ran across an article on Epstein-Barr/CFS in a health food magazine written by a physician. Then I was amazed and delighted to learn that the physician's office wasn't too far from me. He offered me not only superb medical care, but concern and compassion as well. He put me on a comprehensive treatment program which included a sugar-free special diet and the antiyeast medication, nystatin. He also gave me daily injections of vitamin B and I supplemented my diet with vitamins and minerals.

"I slowly began to improve and the changes did not occur overnight. But I gradually turned the corner back toward the living. I've continued to read and study about CFS and yeast infections and the many different factors which can cause it. I've had all of my mercury amalgams removed and I've changed my diet so that I eat most organically grown vegetables and whole grains, a limited amount of fruits and a small amount of fish, fowl and meats.

"One thing I've learned is that there's no hope of ever controlling CFS unless the underlying yeast condition is treated. I'm in control again, but all of my priorities have changed. I no longer sleep in the office because I have so much work to do. I also have a good laugh every day."

Alberta resigned her Army commission which she held for many years and opened a private law practice in 1994. Although I haven't heard from her recently, in 1998 I learned from her secretary that she has ten lawyers working under her supervision and enjoys excellent health.

JUDITH

"I first became ill in 1970 following a bad case of flu. Instead of recovering normally, I continued to deteriorate, and the unexplained illness kept me in bed for six months. A string of doctors insisted that since my tests were all normal, I was not physically ill. They suggested psychiatric care. Eventually, I returned, rather shakily, to work. I assumed that this strange episode was just a fluke, a one-time event that I could put behind me.

"It was not to be. The illness that had no name returned again and again, throwing my life into utter disarray. Eighteen years passed as I became sick and then well and then sick again. I spent a lot of time trapped in bed, wondering how such a devastating disease could be totally dismissed by the medical profession.

"... I weighed about 80 pounds. My digestive processes—not to mention my mental faculties—seemed to have shut down for good. I was in severe pain, and my allergies exploded to include almost every chemical imaginable. Exposure to ordinary things like books, newspapers, TV, or plastic bags sent my brain reeling. A constant 'brain fog' dogged me.

"And then, very unexpectedly, I was diagnosed at last—not by seeing a doctor, but by talking on the phone to a nutritionist. *I learned that I probably had a severe yeast-related health problem.* Not long after the diagnosis was confirmed, I looked into my mouth. To my horror I saw a veritable rain forest of white gummy growth hanging in strings off the edges of my tongue. The mystery malady was solved at last.

"In addition to the usual culprits of birth control pills, antibiotics and moldy environment, another factor caused me to become severely fungus-ridden. For the many years I worked as an artist and printmaker, I practically bathed in dangerous chemicals. There's no doubt in my mind that these toxic substances and not any virus, was the root cause of my illness.

"With the problem identified I was able to assemble and (allergies permitting) read some important books on the subject. A friend brought me your 1986 book *The Yeast Connection.* What a relief to see it all spelled out for me! I had a real illness. It wasn't psychological, and it could be treated.

"I was by this time more dead than alive. A skeleton with a heartbeat. When I became allergic, even to my little Berkeley room, I was brought home, presumably to die. Fate intervened, and almost by accident I was put in contact with a doctor who understood this condition and how to treat it: Vincent Marinkovich, M.D. Under his care I began a program with diet and antifungal drugs.

"One day, more than a year after I began treatment, I embarked on a great adventure. I left the house under my own power and went for a walk. A very slow walk to be sure, but most exciting. I was out in the world again!

"Personal experience has convinced me that so-called chronic fatigue syndrome is basically a disease of toxicity, frequently involving candidiasis. To tell my experiences, and to provide help to others, I wrote *Immune Dysfunction—Winning My Battle Against Toxins, Illness & the Medical Establishment.**

---

*You can read more about Judith Lopez's fascinating story on line at *www.bookzone.com,* or you can order her book from Millpond Press, P. O. Box 2524, Mill Valley, CA 94942.

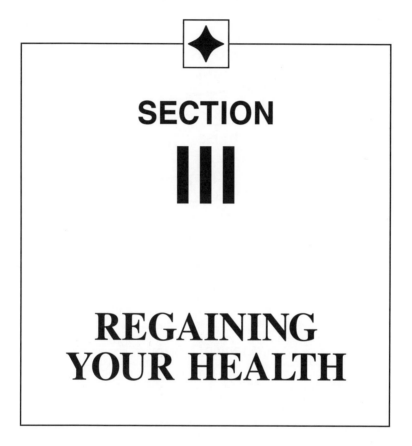

SECTION

III

**REGAINING
YOUR HEALTH**

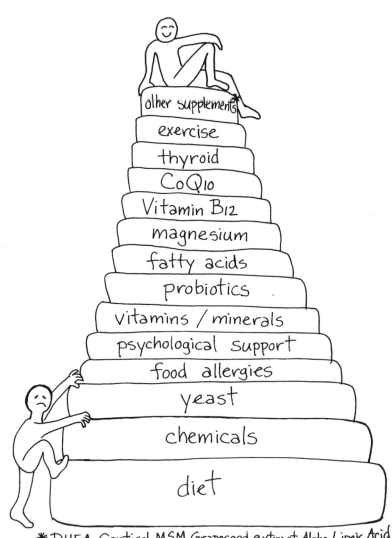

An Overview

I f you're sick and tired, you may resemble an overloaded camel. To regain your health, look good, feel good and enjoy life, you'll need to unload "many bundles of straw." This may take months—even a year or more. But then your camel will be off and running.

The first step in regaining your health is cleaning up your diet and getting rid of junk food. While you're doing this, get rid of the pollutants in your home. You'll, of course, need to make lifestyle changes, obtain sufficient rest and work with your health professional. Then, do simple detective work which will enable you to track down and avoid foods that cause allergic reactions.

Next, because the pesky yeast *Candida albicans* gets out of control in people with weakened immune systems, take steps to control candida. These include avoiding sugar and other simple carbohydrates and taking prescription and nonprescription anti-yeast medication.

You'll also need to take nutritional supplements, including flaxseed oil and other essential fatty acids, vitamins and minerals, including magnesium and zinc. Other nutritional supplements will also help you, including vitamin B_{12} and CoQ_{10}. Because you, like many other people with persistent fatigue may be low in thyroid, you'll need to work with your health professional to find out if you need thyroid supplements.

You'll also need psychological help from your spouse or other significant persons in your life, and from a support group. Also as your strength returns, you'll need to gradually increase your exercise.

The pictures and notes in this section will help you get started. You'll find additional information in Sections IV of this book.*

The Importance of Multiple Therapies

In the front of this book, in "A Special Message to the Reader," I included one of my favorite illustrations—the overloaded camel. This illustration shows that tired people, including those with CFS, develop their health problems from many different causes. And in my discussion of the "yeast connection" and the skepticism and controversy that has surrounded it, I referred to an article by William E. Dismukes and associates which was featured in the *New England Journal of Medicine* in 1990.

The investigators evaluated a group of women with vaginitis who complained of fatigue and many other symptoms. When they failed to respond to a single therapeutic intervention, oral nystatin, they concluded that the symptoms were not yeast related. (See page 163)

Although in this book I've discussed many of the causes and therapies for people who are tired - so tired, other therapies may be needed.

The Fall 1999 issue of *Update,*† a publication of the Functional Medicine Research Center, described the response of two patients to multimodality therapy. Here's information about one of these patients, a 42-year-old Caucasian female.

Her symptoms included severe fatigue, joint pains and stiffness, muscle pains, almost constant headache and poor mental processing. Laboratory studies were carried out and the fol-

---

*If, in spite of this treatment program, you continue to be troubled by insomnia, depression and muscle pains, your physician may prescribe medications which will help relieve these and other symptoms.

†Functional Medicine Research Center, P.O. Box 1729, Gig Harbor, Washington 98335.

lowing tentative diagnoses were made: "Probable chronic fatigue syndrome, multiple food hypersensitivities, fibromyalgia-like syndrome and intestinal candidiasis."

An 8-week treatment program included prescription and nonprescription medications and nutritional supplements. Here are some of the therapies which were used.

An elimination/challenge diet was carried out which showed dramatic allergic reactions with reintroduction of wheat, dairy and coffee. Nonprescription medications included glucosamine sulfate, St. John's wort, Boswellia, garlic, multivitamins, vitamin B_{12} injections, UltraInflamX,™ and Mitochondrial Resuscitate (MR). Prescription medications included sodium levothyroxin and nystatin, which was prescribed at the four-week follow up.

The patient gradually improved and at a 4-month follow up *Update* said, "Further improvement of symptoms—10% of original intensity is reported. Patient feels 'energetic and good' most of the time. Candida antibodies have normalized."

My Comments: This patient gave a long, long history of health disorders, including gall bladder disease, recurrent allergies, vaginitis and ureteral stricture. She had also been exposed to formaldehyde/organic solvents at her workplace. *This report showed that a comprehensive diagnostic and therapeutic approach is needed to help many patients with these problems.*

Clean Up Your Diet

The diet* of Americans has changed dramatically since pioneer days. We live in a "fast-food" society and eat processed and packaged foods which contain sugar, food coloring, flavors, chemicals, additives and pesticides. We drink beverages that are loaded with sugar, phosphates, caffeine, food colors, aspartame and other additives.

Although changing your diet won't be easy, you'll improve significantly—even dramatically—when you make the changes suggested on the next few pages.

Avoid:

Foods and drinks containing sugar, and those containing food colors, phosphates, aspartame and other additives and flavors.

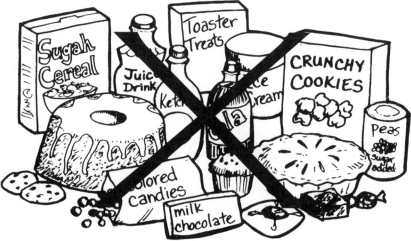

---

*You'll find a further discussion of diet in Section IV.

Processed and packaged foods containing hydrogenated or partially hydrogenated vegetable oils and other "bad fats."

Eat:

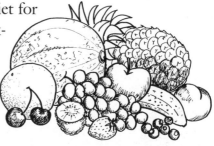

Eat tomatoes, onions, celery, cabbage, cauliflower and asparagus. Also, try some of the many other vegetables which are available, including snow peas, radishes, peppers, jicama, kale, brussels sprouts, cucumbers, okra and bell pepper.

And if you aren't struggling with weight problems, rotate baked Irish potatoes and sweet potatoes and more legumes.

After you've been on the diet for about three weeks, you may experiment with fruits if you're doing well. But do it cautiously, with only a small portion once a day. Then you can feel your way along.

You may also try whole grains in limited amounts—don't overload. Also diversify your diet with the grain alternatives amaranth and quinoa. (For recipes see *The Yeast Connection Cookbook*.)

Fish. Choose ocean fish, including cod, haddock, flounder, grouper, pollock and snapper, as they're less apt to contain toxic pollutants, if they're caught away from the shore. Also shrimp, lobster, crab and oyster. (Take precautions to lessen the chance they're contaminated.)

Meats. Wild game, chicken, beef, pork, lamb—especially lean meats from animals who haven't been treated with hormones.

Buy "expeller pressed" vegetable oils which are organically grown and unrefined. They're available in health food stores and in some supermarkets. Olive oil is also an excellent oil to use in cooking.

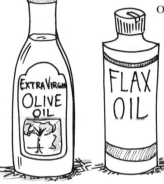

Get flax oil and/or organically grown flax seeds from your health food store.

Look for "organically produced," chemically uncontaminated meats, fruits, vegetables and grains. (See Section V, page 281.)

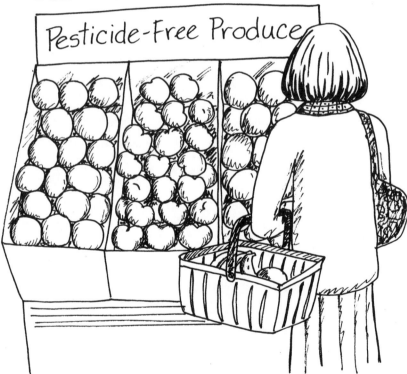

Be an informed consumer. Read magazines and books you'll find in your health food stores, including *Alive, Better Nutri-*

tion, Delicious, Health Confidential and *Let's Live*. Also subscribe to:

- ✦ *Consumers' Research Magazine* by Consumers' Research Inc., 800 Maryland Ave., N.E., Washington, DC 20002. E-mail: Crmag@aol.com. 888-265-4322 (toll free)
- ✦ *Nutrition Action Healthletter,* Center for Science in the Public Interest, 1875 Connecticut Ave., N.W., Washington, DC 20009-5728. E-mail: CIRC@cspinet.org. Webpage: www.cspinet.org. 202-332-9110. ($24)
- ✦ *Bottom Line Health,* Box 451, Greenwich, CT 06863
- ✦ *NOHA News* (Nutrition for Optimal Health Association), www.nutrition.4health.org 847-604-3258 ($10).

Clean Up Your Home Environment

Everyone knows that chemical pollutants* in the air, soil, food and water are adversely affecting us and our families. Yet, you may be surprised to learn that indoor air pollutants may be bothering you more than those you're exposed to outdoors.

Some years ago Theron Randolph,[1] a pioneer Chicago internist, allergist and specialist in environmental medicine, warned:

"While it is true that outdoor air pollution is a significant source of exposure, *a far greater threat is posed by the presence of indoor . . . air pollution. . . . Many household products give off noxious fumes. Indoor air pollution is particularly dangerous because exposure is so constant.*"

During the past 30 years, Randolph and several hundred physicians and other professionals in the American Academy of Environmental Medicine have been studying and treating patients with chronic health disorders related to chemical overload. And they have found that by lightening this load, many patients with puzzling and persistent health problems improve.

The person with environmentally induced illness (EI) or multiple chemical sensitivity (MCS) and their physicians who are working to help them have faced much of the same sort of

---

*You'll find a comprehensive discussion of chemicals in our environment and the hazards they pose in Section IV.

skepticism and hostility as those who have been working to bring CFS into the medical mainstream. Yet, happily, the situation seems to be changing.*

A good friend and courageous crusader, Agnes Jonas, a Connecticut woman, has written thousands of letters and knocked on the doors of senators and representatives in her state saying, "Please stop, look and listen. Countless people are being made ill by environmental pollutants." Because of her wonderful work, Ms. Jonas is now a member of the Advisory Board of the International Health Foundation.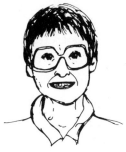

Here are a few suggestions which will help you get started and learn more about chemical pollutants.

1. Don't smoke, and don't let people smoke in your home. People in homes where others are smoking experience *twice* as many respiratory infections as individuals in smoke-free homes, and such infections set up a vicious cycle of other health problems.

2. Don't spray insecticides inside or outside of your home, and keep your windows closed on the days your neighbors spray their houses.

3. Try to bring about changes in your workplace. If your office is making you sick, bring information to your employer or seek a job in a less polluted environment.

4. Get a copy of the superb book by Lynn Lawson, *Staying Well in a Toxic World*. This book is not only authoritative

*For names of physicians in your area interested in EI or MCS, send a $5 donation or a self-addressed, stamped envelope to AAEM, 7701 E. Kellogg, Suite 625, Wichita, KS 67207.

and carefully documented, it's as readable as a paperback novel. Even if you aren't bothered by chemical sensitivities, call or write Lynnword Press, P. O. Box 1732, Evanston, IL 60201, 1-847-866-9630. You can also search the internet.

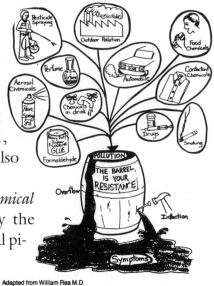

5. Get a copy of the book *Chemical Sensitivity** (Vol I–IV) by the physician and environmental pioneer, William Rea, M.D. According to Rea, your resistance resembles a rain

Adapted from William Rea M.D. Used with permission.

barrel and chemicals in your environment are like pipes draining into the barrel. When you're exposed to many chemicals, your barrel overflows and symptoms develop.

Sound Advice from Ann Landers

The Newsletter of MCS: Health & Environment[†] included this advice from Ann Landers:

"Speak up readers. The consumer is king."

Ann made these comments in responding to a woman from Ontario with multiple chemical sensitivity. Here are excerpts from Ann's column.

---

*For more information about these books or Dr. Rea's other publications, call 800-428-2343.

†Newsletter of MCS: Health & Environment, edited by Lynn Lawson, 1404 Judson Ave., Evanston, IL 60201. e-mail: linnword@aol.com.

"I have become so sensitive to so many chemicals that I am like that canary in the coal mine. If I sit next to a person for a minute, I will react to his or her laundry detergent, perfume, antiperspirant, hair spray, and so on. I'm also affected by car exhaust fumes and must wear a mask to go for a drive or a walk outside. In order to create a livable environment for myself, I had to remove every chemical in my home.

". . . My plea is to manufacturers who put toxic chemicals, such as perfumes, in their products when they are not necessary. The only products I use to clean my house are Borax, baking soda and vinegar. Those do the job just as well as those high priced brand name chemical cleaners. Please, Ann, tell them to stop adding all that stuff before all of us become incapacitated."

Ann responded,

"Your letter will be greatly appreciated by readers who have the same problem. Meanwhile, the sale of Borax, baking soda and vinegar is sure to increase because of what you wrote. We've been using all of those in my home for a long time. I learned about their effectiveness from my mother. Many readers complained about magazines that inserted highly perfumed ads for fragrances, and I see that the practice has decreased. Speak up readers. The consumer really is king."

Sound Advice From England

In an article entitled "Multiple Chemical Sensitivity—A personal experience," in the spring 2000 issue of the *Allergy Newsletter* published by Action Against Allergy (AAA), Maxima Skelton* said,

---

*You can find more information about Skelton and her observations and publications on the internet, www.healthyhouse.co.uk.

"Through my work I have talked to hundreds of chemically sensitive people and others who are searching for the cause of their symptoms. . . . Many are sensitive to chemical treatments on carpets and upholstered furniture and furnishings. Most modern homes are very toxic. The pollution level inside a house is many times higher than in the air outside, even in a polluted area.

"The most common chemicals found in a house are formaldehyde and hydrocarbons. . . Other chemicals which create a problem for chemically sensitive people are terpenes, ethylene and VOCs (volatile organic compounds). Volatile organic compounds—toluene, xylene, hexanes, benzene—evaporate into the air we breathe and cause many problems.

"Other products to be aware of are chlorinated water, pesticides, insecticides, fragrances and perfumes, deodorants, cleaning products and detergents, dry cleaning solvents, anaesthetics and prescribed medications, heavy metals (particularly mercury and dental fillings), artificial colourings, flavouring and preservatives in foods, drink and drugs . . ."

In discussing more practical solutions, Skelton included these recommendations "for anyone wishing to live in a less polluted environment."

"Remove as many synthetic materials from the home and workplace as possible, this includes vinyl, plastic, foam rubber, chipped board and possibly pine. Remove toxic cleaning chemicals and polishes, synthetic soaps, detergents and perfumed products.

"Use a water purifier to remove chlorine and pollutants from the water or boil all drinking water to remove the chlorine.

"Use nontoxic paints and varnishes, unperfumed detergents, natural soaps and shampoos, untreated cotton and wool bedding.

"Do not use synthetic materials or chemically treated materials either for bedding or for clothing; do not have clothes or bedding dry cleaned; do not use detergents or fabric softeners that contain formaldehyde."

Skelton advised people to use cane, wood, leather, wool and other natural fibers for furniture and furnishings; to remove gas appliances and use electricity or put the gas furnace in the garage away from the main living area of the home. She urged people to cover floors with cotton rugs because carpets are often treated with insecticides and fungicides.

She also pointed out that many sensitive people are affected by computers, televisions or other products made of hard plastic and are sensitive to electrical and magnetic fields. And in concluding her remarks, she said,

> *"Given the many chemicals we're exposed to on a daily basis, it's hardly surprising that the number of people suffering from chronic chemical sensitivity is increasing . . . Chemical sensitivity is a disease of the late 20th Century. We need to look back and remember how our grandparents lived and adopt a few of their routines."*[2]

REFERENCES

1. Randolph, T.G. and Moss, R.W., *An Alternative Approach to Allergies,* New York: Harper and Row, 1989, p. 50.
2. Action Against Allergy, P.O. Box 278, Twickenham, Middlesex, TWI 4QQ. E-mail: AAA@ actionagainst allergy.freeserve.co.uk.

Control Yeasts

Prescription Medications

Chronic fatigue is especially apt to be yeast related if you've taken repeated or prolonged courses of amoxicillin, Ceclor or the tetracyclines during infancy, childhood and adolescence, or since you've become an adult. These drugs knock out friendly germs while they're knocking out enemies.

Candida yeasts are *not* affected by antibiotics so they multiply and raise large families. These yeasts put out toxins that weaken the immune system. So you may experience repeated infections. Each infection is treated with antibiotics, so a vicious cycle develops.*

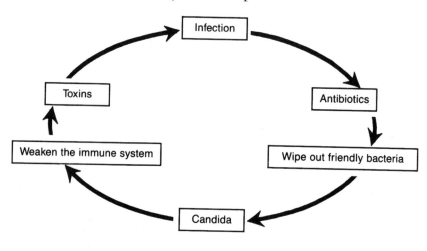

---

*See also Section IV.

Other Factors

Yeast overgrowth also can be caused by other factors, including:

+ A diet rich in sugar and other simple carbohydrates that promote yeast overgrowth.
+ Hormonal changes associated with the normal menstrual cycle.
+ Birth control pills.
+ Pregnancy.
+ Steroids, taken by pill, injection or inhalation.
+ Genital irritations and abrasions.
+ Re-infection from your sexual partner.
+ Diabetes.

The yeast infection in your genital area also may be related to wearing jockey shorts or nylon underwear.

How Superficial Yeast Infections Can Cause Chronic Fatigue

A yeast infection in one part of your body can cause symptoms in other parts of your body in several different ways.

Immune System Disturbances

Studies by Japanese researchers at the University of Tokyo show that *Candida albicans* puts out high and low molecular weight toxins that can weaken your immune system.[1,2] Other researchers have also noted the relationship of intestinal and vaginal yeast infections to immunological problems.[3]

Absorption of Food Antigens—and Toxins

Based on clinical and research studies by many different observers, candida overgrowth in your intestine may create what has been called a "leaky gut." Toxins and food allergens* may then pass through this membrane and go to other parts of your body, making you feel "sick all over."

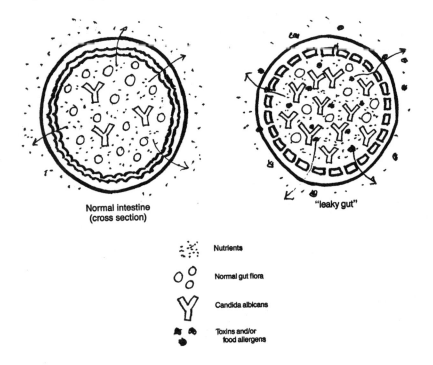

Normal intestine
(cross section)

"leaky gut"

Nutrients

Normal gut flora

Candida albicans

Toxins and/or
food allergens

Allergies to Candida

According to James Brodsky, M.D.:

"There is much evidence to suggest that C. albicans is one of the most allergenic microbes. Both immediate and delayed

*The role of probiotics in the management of food allergies was reported in the *Journal of Allergy and Clinical Immunology*, 99:179–85; 1997.

hypersensitivity reactions to candida are very common in the adult population."

The Diagnosis of a Yeast-Related Disorder

How does your physician make a diagnosis? How does she find out why you're troubled by fatigue, headache, depression or other symptoms? She bases her conclusions on:

+ Your history or story. This includes not only your main complaints, but also symptoms or events in your past history that are important.
+ Your physical examination. This should include an overall look at your body, along with closer examination of your skin, eyes, heart, lungs and other parts of your body.
+ Laboratory examinations, other tests and x-rays.*

It's usually harder to diagnose a yeast-related problem than a fractured leg, pneumonia, or many other disorders. And a physical examination and tests do not provide your physician with all of the information she needs to make a diagnosis.

Nevertheless, if you're "tired—so tired" you should go to a physician for a checkup. If your physical examination and "routine" laboratory tests are normal, and you make a high score on the yeast questionnaire, a yeast-connected disorder is possible or probable. The diagnosis is confirmed by noting your response to a simple but *comprehensive* treatment program. Such a program features a sugar-free special diet and prescription and nonprescription antifungal medications.

---

*Adapted from *The Yeast Connection Handbook,* 2000 edition, Professional Books, Jackson, TN. For information about ordering this book see www.candida-yeast.com/bookstore.

REFERENCES

1. Iwata, K. and Yamamoto, Y., "Glycoprotein Toxins Produced by Candida albicans," Proceedings of the Fourth International Conference on the Mykoses, June 1977, PAHO Scientific Publication, No. 356.

2. Iwata, K. and Uchida, K., "Cellular Immunity in Experimental Fungal Infections in Mice," Mykosen Suppl., 1, 72–81, 1978.

3. Miles, M.R., Olsen, and Rogers, A., "Recurrent Vaginal Candidiasis: Importance of an intestinal reservoir," *JAMA,* 238:1836–1837, October 28, 1977.

Track Down Hidden Food Allergies

Systemic and nervous symptoms caused by food allergies have been described by dozens of professionals during the past several decades. Yet, this relationship is often overlooked by physicians and other professionals. Here's why.

*Hidden, masked or delayed-onset food allergies (and/or adverse food reactions) cannot be positively identified by allergy skin tests or laboratory tests. Yet, they can often be identified by carefully designed, properly executed elimination diets.** Any dietary ingredient can provoke nervous symptoms, including milk, food colors, additives, sugar, wheat, corn, egg, chocolate, yeast and citrus.

Here are some of the questions people ask about these diets and my answers.

Q: How do I find out if my fatigue and other symptoms are caused by something I'm eating?

A: You carry out an elimination diet† avoiding many of your favorite foods.

Q: What will I look for? How will I know these foods bother me?

A: If you're sensitive to the foods you avoid, your symptoms will improve or disappear when you stop eating them. And they'll return when you eat them again.‡

---

*Electroacupuncture or muscle testing by a knowledgeable health professional may also help you suspect foods that are causing adverse reactions. See pp. 264–269.

†You'll find detailed instructions for carrying out this diet in Section V.

‡If you have had asthma or experienced swelling or other serious allergic reactions, get the help and consultation of your physicians before carrying out this diet.

Q: What do I do first?

A: Discuss the diet with other family members. Ask for their cooperation.

Q: How long does it take to do the diet?

A: The elimination part of the diet lasts about a week, or until you show a convincing improvement in your symptoms. Then, the second week, eat the foods you've eliminated— one food per day—and see if your symptoms return.

Q: Please tell me more about the diet.

A: Pick a convenient time.

Don't try it during a holiday or when you're visiting. Before beginning the diet keep a symptom and food diary for three days.

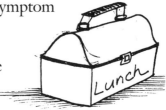

Continue the diary while you're eliminating foods and while you're eating them again.

If you eat away from home, take your food with you.

Q: If I've identified several foods that bother me and am continuing to experience symptoms, what should I do?

A: You'll have to do more detective work. Here are my suggestions.

1. Consider the possibility that chemical contaminants in or on your foods are causing problems.
2. Remember that any food can cause symptoms, including beef, apple, chicken, potato, peanut and/or other foods.

To identify sensitivity to these foods try the Caveman Diet for a week.

On this diet, you avoid any food you eat more than once a week.

Here's good news. As you control the overgrowth of *Candida albicans* in your digestive tract and your immune system improves, your food sensitivities will lessen and may disappear.

What You Can Eat or Drink on the Diet

+ Any vegetable but corn and any fruit but orange (or other food that you consume on a daily basis)
+ Any meat but bacon, sausage, hot dogs and luncheon meat
+ Oats, rice, barley and the grain alternatives, amaranth and quinoa
+ Unprocessed nuts
+ Water (preferably bottled water)

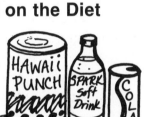

What You'll Need to Avoid on the Diet

+ Oranges*
+ Soft drinks, Kool-Aid and punches
+ Wheat
+ Corn
+ Chocolate
+ Food colors, additives and flavors
+ Milk
+ Simple sugars, including cane sugar, beet sugar, corn syrup, maple syrup and honey
+ Yeast
+ Processed and packaged foods

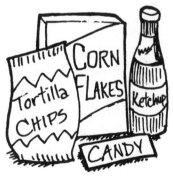

---

*Or any fruit you consume several times a week.

Psychological Factors

I disagree strongly with professionals who say, "There's nothing really wrong with people who complain of being tired. They develop symptoms because life isn't going to suit them—or from other psychological causes." In my opinion, such critics are *not* listening to their patients or reading the medical literature. If they did they'd realize that viral infections, food allergies and chemical sensitivities are common causes of people feeling persistently tired. And if they would open their minds and their hearts, they'd realize that repeated antibiotics, high sugar diets and steroids result in the overgrowth of *Candida albicans* and the role it plays in making people tired and feel "sick all over."*

Psychological factors *are* important in people with every health problem, whether it's heart disease, arthritis or the chronic fatigue syndrome (CFS). Such factors have been documented to weaken the immune system. For example, studies I've read in medical journals show that T-lymphocytes (the cells which protect people from viral and other infections) were significantly reduced following the death of a spouse or a child.

On a more favorable note, the observations of the late Norman Cousins show that the immune system can be strengthened and recovery from many illnesses accelerated by laughter and other psychological nutrients.

During the 1980s, I visited Mr. Cousins in his office at

---

*To obtain further information, physicians (and other health professionals) can read a 24-page booklet, *A Special Message to the Health Professional*. A copy of this booklet can be obtained from IHF, Box 3494, Jackson, TN 38303. A donation of $10 is requested.

UCLA. During our fascinating conversations he told me of his work with groups of patients with arthritis, cancer and other chronic, disabling and painful illnesses. He said, "I always tell them jokes. After the third joke I've seen them laughing so hard they have to hold their sides." Then when my session is completed, I ask, "How many of you are still hurting as much as you were when you walked into this room?" No hands were raised.

Surgeon, writer and lecturer Bernie Siegel, who published a number of books dealing with the importance of psychological support, stresses the importance of the link between mind and body. He urges people with chronic diseases to learn to have fun. Specific suggestions included reading humorous books and going to light, entertaining movies. He also urged people to play games, tell jokes to their friends. He also said that you can have fun with coloring books and do anything else that will bring out the child inside you.

In his book *Maximum Immunity* published over a decade ago, Michael A. Weiner, Ph.D., described a study carried out on cadets at West Point to see how psychological factors influenced their susceptibility to infectious mononucleosis.

"Cadets were selected at the beginning of the study who were free of the antibody for the Epstein-Barr Virus. . . During their stay at the academy, some of the young men developed the Epstein-Barr Virus antibody; but only some of these actually developed mononucleosis. The others remained symptom free, indicating that they had better resistance. The cadets who became sick with infectious mononucleosis were generally found to have experienced greater academic pressure and to have shown poorer academic performance than the resistant group of cadets."

Weiner cited another study of a group of students in which "it was found that failure, social isolation and unresolved role crisis was often associated with respiratory infections. The more serious the sickness, the more likely it was that stressful situations had occurred during the preceding year."[1]

What do these observations mean? *Psychological stress can play a part in making you more susceptible to illnesses of many types and psychological support can help you get well.* In talking to my patients about such support, I like to use the term "psychological vitamins." Here are some of them.

+ You need caring, empathetic people to encourage you, work with you and help you. Included, of course, would be your spouse or companion who lives with you, or a relative or best friend. It could also include a professional who understands your illness and works to help you. Support groups consisting of people who are experiencing similar problems can also help.

+ You need to be noticed, praised and encouraged. You need smiles, touching, holding, patting and petting. Physical contact stimulates the release of endorphins, a chemical which lessens anxiety and pain.

In his book *Touching,* Ashley Montagu told of scientific studies with rats. "The more handling and petting the rats received, the better they did in laboratory situations."[2]

+ In spite of your health problems, you need to have a feeling of accomplishment. Whether you work in an office or at home, or whether you're a salesman on the road, you need to enjoy the work you're doing. You need to feel that it makes a difference. You need to feel appreciated.

To summarize. Although psychological factors are rarely *the* cause of chronic fatigue, they can play a part in weakening your immune system and contributing to your health problems. Conversely, love, laughter, praise, touching and other psychological nutrients can help you regain your health and get your life back on track.

REFERENCES

1. Weiner, M.A., *Maximum Immunity,* Houghton and Mifflin, New York, 1986.

2. Montagu, A., *Touching: The Human Significance of the Skin,* Albany University Press, New York, 1971.

Vitamin/Mineral Supplements

I take these supplements and recommend them for my friends, family and patients. Although I freely admit that if you:

+ eat a "truly" good diet, which features lots of vegetables, as well as whole grains, fruits, beans, nuts, seeds, some fish and/or animal products; and, if the foods are organically grown on nutritionally rich soil
+ avoid or sharply limit the "junk foods" (which are refined and processed or contain hydrogenated or partially hydrogenated fats and oils) and beverages loaded with sugar, phosphates, food coloring and additives
+ aren't exposed to environmental chemicals including traffic fumes, tobacco, insecticides and other home chemicals

you would not need nutritional supplements. *BUT, no person on this planet today, including people with fatigue, meet these requirements. Accordingly, I recommend them.*

During the past 15 years, nutritional biochemist Jeffrey S. Bland, Ph.D., (in his articles, books, lectures and audio tape presentations) has emphasized the importance of consuming more than the RDA (recommended daily allowances) of the micronutrients if we wish to enjoy optimal health throughout our lives.

In discussing the importance of nutrition with me recently, Donald R. Davis, Ph.D. (a long-time associate of the late Roger

J. Williams, Ph.D.), Biochemical Institute, University of Texas, Austin 78712 said,

> "Americans, on average, get well over half of their calories from three kinds of nutrient-depleted 'foods' that are never fed in similar quantities to prized animals of any kind. These three kinds of foods are (1) added, refined sugars, (2) added fats and oils, and (3) white flour and white rice which have had their nutrient-rich germ and bran removed. Combined, they amount to a large daily cookie of about 1500 calories for every American. Few Americans realize this fact.
>
> "By far, the best way that Americans can improve their nutrition and lessen their risk for many kinds of health problems is to greatly reduce their consumption of cookie ingredients and replace them with what nature provides for us:
>
> "Fruits, melons and sweet vegetables instead of added sugars found in soft drinks, candies and many other sugared products. Fruit juices of the unusual 100% type are far superior to sweetened beverages, but whole fruits are nutritionally preferable to juices.
>
> "Nuts, oily seeds, avocados, olives, coconut, soy and milk products instead of oils (any kind), butter, margarine, shortening and mayonnaise.
>
> "Whole—or mostly whole—grain products, instead of white flour and rice."*

Whole foods are also important for your children. As you know, children are "parent watchers," and if you "turn up your nose" at broccoli and carrots, they'll do the same.

In November 1999, at Georgetown University's conference, *ADHD: Causes and Possible Solutions,*† Dr. Davis presented a position paper entitled "Nutritional Deficiency in American Children." Here's a brief excerpt of his comments.

---

*Personal communication, April 2000.

†For a two-page summary of this conference send a $3 donation and SASE to IHF, Box 3494, Jackson, TN 38303.

"Whole foods were nearly the only kind of food available during our genetic evolution. The strong merits of whole foods derive from a simple fact: They consist of once-living cells that required for their growth and function a complex mixture of the same vitamins, minerals, trace minerals, amino acids, fatty acids, carbohydrates and other substances that our cells need for their growth and healthy function . . . When children and others replaced natural diets of whole foods with the equivalent of a large daily cookie of 1000 to 1500 calories, or sometimes more, we should not be surprised to find numerous problems. . . And we should keep open to the possibility that such unnatural diets may contribute to behavior problems such as ADHD.

"The outstanding nutritional value of whole foods is illustrated by NutriCircles(R) diagrams created by Dr. Williams and me in 1977. The diagrams are available on personal computers for over 2000 foods."*

In a Utopian world you'd be consuming a wide variety of nutritious foods grown organically on nonchemically polluted soil. You'd also be breathing clean air at home and in your community and you would not be exposed to tobacco smoke, lawn chemicals, diesel fumes and other toxic substances.

BUT, in the real world of the 2000s, I recommend insurance vitamins and minerals. Those I recommend for my adult patients with yeast-connected health problems and/or CFS contain:

Vitamin A, 5,000-10,000 IU	Calcium, 500 mg
Beta-carotene, 15,000 IU	Magnesium, 500 mg
Vitamin B1, 25–100 mg daily	Inositol, 100 mg
Vitamin B2, 25–50 mg daily	Citrus bioflavonoids, 100 mg
Niacinamide, 100–150 mg daily	PABA, 50 mg
Pantothenic acid, 100–500 mg daily	Zinc, 15–30 mg

---

*Copies of NutriCircles® are available free on the internet at www.cm.utexas.edu/williams. Click on NutriCircles® food diagrams.

Vitamin B$_6$, 25–100 mg daily
Folic acid, 200–800 mcg
Vitamin B$_{12}$, 100 mcg
Biotin, 300 mcg
Choline(Bitartrate), 100 mg
Vitamin C[†], 1000–3,000 mg
Vitamin D, 400–800 IU
Vitamin E, 400–600 IU

Copper, 1–2 mg
Iron,[*] 15–20 mg
Manganese, 20 mg
Selenium, 100–200 mcg
Chromium, 200 mcg
Molybdenum, 100 mcg
Vanadium, 25 mcg
Boron, 1 mg

When these supplements are prescribed by a knowledgeable professional, the amounts may vary considerably from those I've outlined, and his or her experience, expertise and clinical judgment will override my recommendations.

Support for the Use of Vitamin/Mineral Supplements

Although the use of vitamin/mineral supplements continues to be "controversial," there is increasing interest and support coming from many sides. According to James S. Goodwin, M.D. and Michael R. Tangum, M.D., the Center on Aging, University of Texas Medical Branch (Galveston), in their commentary published in a major medical journal

"Throughout the 20th century American academic medicine has resisted the concept that supplementation with micronutrients might have health benefits. This resistance is evidenced in several ways:

---

[*]Iron supplements are given only to individuals who are anemic or who are losing blood. (See also pages 345–346.)

[†]Based on the observations of Linus Pauling, Ph.D. and Robert Cathcart, M.D., much larger doses may benefit patients with serious medical problems. The appropriate dosage is determined by the "bowel tolerance test."

1. By the uncritical acceptance of news of toxicity, such as the belief that vitamin C supplements cause kidney stones;
2. By the angry, scornful tone used in discussions of micronutrient supplementation in the leading textbooks of medicine;
3. By ignoring evidence for possible efficacy of a micronutrient supplement such as the use of vitamin E for intermittent claudication.

"Part of the resistance stems from the fact that the potential benefits of micronutrients were advanced by outsiders, who took their message directly to the public, and part from the fact that the concept of a deficiency disease did not fit in well with prevailing medical paradigms, particularly the germ theory. Similar factors might be expected to color the response of academic medicine to any alternative treatment."

In their fascinating article, Goodwin and Tangum compared the resistance of the medical establishment to micronutrient supplements to the problems Galileo experienced in his struggle with the Catholic church.

"Galileo's crime was not his propounding a heliocentric universe; it was that he wrote in Italian—directly to the public. Previous scientists wrote in Latin, limiting their audience to other scholars.

". . . The 17th Century church represented the intellectual establishment . . . Galileo was punished not for writing heresy, not for threatening paradigms, but for bypassing the intellectual establishment in taking his exciting ideas directly to the people."

In the conclusion of their article these physicians said,

"There are only 3 important questions when evaluating a potential treatment. *Does it work? What are the adverse effects? How much does it cost?* Ideally, issues such as the theory underlying the treatment or the guild to which the proponents of the treatment belong should be irrelevant to the fundamental questions of efficacy, toxicity, and cost. The history of the response of academic medicine to micronutrient supplementation suggests that we have not attained that ideal."[1]

REFERENCE

1. "Battling Quackery, Attitudes About Micronutrient Supplements in American Academic Medicine," James S. Goodwin, M.D. and Michael R. Tangum, M.D., from the Center on Aging, University of Texas Medical Branch (Galveston), Archives of Internal Medicine, Vol. 158, November 9, 1998, pp. 2187–2191.

Probiotics

Probiotics are a group of friendly bacteria that help you stay well. These bacteria, which are found in sugar-free, fruit-free high-quality yogurt, were first identified about 100 years ago. And in 1908, Metchinoff, a Bulgarian, recommended a daily consumption of yogurt because he felt it promoted good health and long life.

During the years since that time preparations of these friendly bacteria have been used by both physicians and nonphysicians to treat complaints ranging from constipation and diarrhea to skin problems.

In introducing their discussion of probiotics the authors of the book *Alternative Medicine* said,

> "Inside each of us live vast numbers of bacteria without which we could not remain in good health . . . There are several thousand billion in each person . . . most of them living in the digestive tract. If they were all placed together the total weight of these 'friendly' bacteria would come to nearly four pounds. . .
>
> "These bacteria . . . perform many important functions in the body . . . however not all of the friendly bacteria perform the same functions. Some being far more useful and plentiful than others. Certain bacteria helps to maintain good health, while others have a definite value in helping us regain health once it's been upset. These dual protective and therapeutic roles help explain why the word probiotics was coined, since it means 'for life.'
>
> "They manufacture some of the B vitamins . . . They manufacture the milk-digesting enzyme, lactase, which helps digest calcium-rich dairy products. They actually produce antibacterial substances which kill or deactivate hostile disease-causing

bacteria. Some bacteria, such as Bifidobacteria and acidophilus have been shown to have anticarcinogenic features. They improve the efficiency of the digestive tract."[1]

During the past 15 years much of the information I've learned about nutrition has come from Jeffery Bland's monthly audio tapes, *Functional Medicine Update*. I've also "picked Jeff's brain" on several occasions. In discussing probiotics with him several years ago, I asked him if he used plain *Lactobacillus acidophilus* or a combination product. In responding, he said,

> "*I think we all recognize that the most important criteria for activity of probiotic substances is there must be an adequate number of live organisms,* they must be reasonably resistant to oxgall (bile), they must be able to adhere to the epithelial membrane. If any one of these three criteria is not met then the activity of the product is limited."[2]

Scientific Support for the Use of Probiotics

In a comprehensive seven-page article researchers from the School of Medicine, University of Washington, Seattle, reviewed the medical literature and described their own observations on the importance of probiotics, including *Lactobacillus acidophilus* and *Bifidobacterium bifidum*. In the conclusion of their article they said,

> "There is now evidence that administration of selected microorganisms is beneficial in the prevention and treatment of certain intestinal and possibly treatment of vaginal, infections. *In an effort to decrease the reliance on antimicrobials, the time has come to carefully explore the therapeutic applications of biotherapeutic agents.*[3] (emphasis added)

Here's a discussion of the use of probiotics in a 1998 book *Chronic Fatigue, Fibromyalgia and Environmental Illness.*

"Since the imbalance of intestinal flora are common among allergy sufferers, Dr. Chaitow stresses the need to restore bowel flora balance with a daily program of probiotics, or the use of friendly or beneficial bacteria that inhabit the intestines under healthy conditions.

"*Lactobacillus acidophilus, Lactobacillus bulgaricus* and the *Bifidobacteria* are the key players in this process," Dr. Chaitow says, "But care must be taken to select the proper strains," he cautions.

"To be effective probiotic supplements should be freeze-dried, contain only the declared and desirable strains of the species and have concentrations of the friendly bacteria of about one billion parts to a gram. They should be kept refrigerated."[4]

In discussing probiotics in his 1998 book, *Biological Treatments for Autism and PDD,* William Shaw, Ph.D., said,

"There are now over 100 brands of beneficial bacteria available in formulations of different kinds. Some of these organisms are grown on dairy products as a source of nutrition while others are dairy free. Because of the sensitivity of most children with autism to the peptides derived from milk, it may be wise to choose a dairy-free brand. . . These products may help to control both yeast and abnormal bacteria such as clostridia in the intestinal tract. . . I recommend the simultaneous use of a probiotic product any time an antifungal drug is used. . . Overgrowth of harmful bacteria may occur unless probiotics are taken simultaneously with prescription and nonprescription antifungal products."[5]

REFERENCES

1. The Burton Goldberg Group, *Alternative Medicine—The Definitive Guide,* Future Medicine Publishing, Tiburon, CA, 1993, pp. 1014–1016.

2. Personal communication.

3. Elmer, G.W., Surawicz, C.M. and McFarland, I.V., "Biothera-

peutic Agents—A neglected modality for the treatment and prevention of selected intestinal and vaginal infections," *JAMA,* 275:870–876, 1996.

4. Goldberg, B. and the editors of *Alternative Medicine Digest, Chronic Fatigue, Fibromyalgia and Environmental Illness,* Future Medicine Publishing, Tiburon, CA, pp. 248–249, Sunflower Press, 1998.

5. Shaw, William, Ph.D., *Biological Treatments for Autism and PDD,* pp. 72–73, 1998.

Essential Fatty Acids

F ats, fats, fats! During the past two decades, newspapers, magazines and TV programs have talked about fats. During the 1980s and on into the 1990s food producers boasted because certain of their products were low in fat or "reduced" in fat, and so on and on.

Then, to make things confusing, Dr. Robert Atkins' bestselling books, which became even more popular during the late 1990s, said in effect, "Don't worry about fats. You can eat bacon, eggs, meat and other fatty foods." Other books and articles have said, "It's not fats that make you fat, it's all of those simple carbohydrates from cereals and breads that are the culprits."

Few people in the media have pointed out that there are good fats as well as bad fats. People need good fats to be healthy. What are these good fats? They're essential fatty acids (EFAs). These fatty acids are found in plants and their seeds, including flax seeds and walnuts. They're also found in the fat of cold water fish, including salmon, mackerel, sardines, tuna and herring. EFAs, like vitamins, cannot be manufactured in your body, so they must be supplied in your diet.

EFAs play many essential roles in the body. Here are a few of them. They store energy and furnish raw material for making prostoglandins and other "short lived" substances required for the second by second regulation of almost all of the tissues of the body. Equally important, they're required for the structure of all cells and all membranes of the body. Because of these diverse functions they're important in preventing health problems of many types, including eczema and other skin disorders, arthritis, heart disease, PMS and chronic fatigue.

There are two general classes of EFAs, one group called the Omega-3 fatty acids and one called the Omega-6 fatty acids.

I first learned about the importance of EFAs in the 1980s from Drs. Sidney Baker, Leo Galland, David Horrobin and Orian Truss, and Laura Stevens, M.S., a Purdue University researcher. Other clinicians and researchers have also emphasized their importance, especially the Omega-3 fatty acids. Here's an explanation for this name.

This long chain of fatty acids begins with a carbon atom with three hydrogen atoms hitched on to it. This is called the CH^3 or Omega end of the molecule. Omega-3 fatty acids have the first double bond on the third carbon atom from the CH^3 end of the molecule. If this sounds complicated to you I can understand, because it's complicated to me as well, because I'm not a biochemist.

Comments by Dr. Sidney M. Baker

In his 1997 book *Detoxification and Healing: The key to optimal health,* Dr. Baker said,

> "Signs of fatty acid problems—basically Omega-3 deficiency—are among the most reliable among the subtle findings in a nutritional assessment of patients. . . . The clues that can be observed on the skin, however, fall into a spectrum in which a theme of dryness is manifested in different ways. They are:
>
> 1. Cracking fingertips—worse in winter.
> 2. Patchy dullness of the skin, especially on the face with a subtle patchy variation in the color of the skin.
> 3. Mixed oily and dry skin which, in cosmetic advertisements, is sometimes called combination skin.
> 4. Chicken skin—which constitutes small, rough bumps on the back of the arms.
> 5. Alligator skin, usually on the lower legs which develop an irregular quilted appearance with dry patches.

6. Stiff, dry, unmanageable, brittle hair.
7. Seborrheic, cracked, cradle cap, dandruff, hair loss.
8. Soft fingernails or brittle fingernails which fray with horizontal splitting.

"These findings usually respond dramatically when a person takes a supplement of Omega-3 oils. Associated symptoms . . . often melt away as the skin signs do. The variety of problems that respond to Omega-3 fatty acid supplementation crosses all the boundaries between system specialties and diseases."[1]

Comments of Dr. Michael Schmidt

In his book *Smart Fats—How Dietary Fats and Oils Affect Mental, Physical and Emotional Intelligence,* Dr. Schmidt said,

"Once we've discarded our notion that all fat is bad we have to establish a new understanding. There are three basic critical points:

✦ "Too much fat in whatever form can lead to disease.
✦ "Too little fat in whatever form can lead to disease.
✦ "The kind of fat and the balance of various fats are the critical features that determine how fats contribute to disease.

"We must remember the brain's major structures have an absolute requirement for fat. Balance of these structural fats appears to be among the most important factors that determine your brains architectural integrity and ultimately, health."[2]

Comments of nutritional counselor Melissa Diane Smith

In an article in the March 1999 *Delicious* magazine, Ms. Smith said that the most important thing to know about EFAs is that a balanced intake of Omega-6 and Omega-3 fatty acids is needed to promote health. And she cited researchers who said,

"The ratio of Omega-6 to Omega-3 fatty acids in the Western diet today is between 10:1 and 21:1, whereas the diet humans evolved on had a ratio of 1:1. . . One of the most important medical findings in recent years is that eating a balance of EFAs brings your diet back into sync with your genes and helps you experience optimal health. . . Omega-3 and Omega-6 work differently in the body . . . when they're in balance they're both very good. When the Omega-6 is in excess they become bad. . .

"Unfortunately, developing a better dietary balance between Omega-3s and Omega-6s isn't easy to do. The source of Omega-3s in the current food supply are scarce to nonexistent, whereas the sources of Omega-6s are ubiquitous. Therefore, we need to reduce dramatically the amount of Omega-6s in our diet as we increase our Omega-3s.

Then she advises, "Other good fats in addition to Omega-3s are monosaturated fats, found in olives, some nuts (macadamias, almonds, peanuts, pecans and cashews), avocados and olive, nut and canola oils. . . Getting back to the delicate balance between Omega-3s and Omega-6s . . . start by avoiding oils with high Omega-6 to Omega-3 ratios, including corn oil, safflower oil, peanut oil, soybean oil, sunflower oil and cottonseed oil. . . Make an oil change. Use cold-pressed extra-virgin olive oil or canola oil in place of Omega-6 oils.

"Finally, eat your veggies—specifically the dark green leafy ones. Especially good sources of Omega-3 EFAs include Romaine lettuce, mesclun mixed greens, arugula, kale, mustard greens and Swiss chard."[3]

EFAs and Chronic Fatigue Syndrome

In a study entitled, "Effect of High Doses of Essential Fatty Acids on the Post-Viral Fatigue Syndrome," P. O. Behan, W. M. H. Behan and D. Horrobin, Departments of Neurology and Pathology at the University of Glasgow, Scotland (Behan and Behan) and Scotia Pharmaceuticals, Guildford, Surrey, England (Horrobin), found that EFAs help people with post-viral fatigue syndrome. Here's an excerpt.

> "Sixty-three adults with the diagnosis of the post-viral fatigue syndrome were enrolled in a double-blind, placebo-controlled study of essential fatty acid therapy. The patients had been ill for from one to three years after an apparently viral infection, suffering from severe fatigue, myalgia and a variety of psychiatric symptoms. . . .
>
> "At 1 month, 74% of the patients on active treatment and 23% of those on placebo assessed themselves as improved over the baseline with the improvement being much greater in the former. At 3 months, the corresponding figures were 85% and 17% (p0.0001) since the placebo group had reverted toward the baseline state while those in the active group showed continued improvement. The essential fatty acids were abnormal at the baseline and corrected by the active treatment. There were no adverse events. *We conclude that essential fatty acids provide a rational, safe and effective treatment for patients with the post-viral fatigue syndrome.*"[4]

In a second article entitled "Essential Fatty Acids, Immunity and Viral Infections," Horrobin stated,

> "There is evidence of a close interrelationship between essential fatty acid (EFA) metabolism and the ability to respond to viral infections."

In this article, he also discussed the importance of a whole series of "cofactors" (including magnesium, biotin, pyridoxine, nicotinic acid, iron, zinc and ascorbic acid) which are required for the normal metabolism of linoleic acid. And he said,

> "All these nutrients must be present in adequate amounts if EFAs are going to have their expected effects."[5]

Here's an anecdotal report which I received in the mail in May 2000.

> "After suffering from recurrent vaginal yeast infections for three years I began an elimination diet about nine months ago. Although I achieved some remission by removing wheat, refined sugars, prepared foods and additives from my diet, I easily relapsed. Then I read Andrew Weil, M.D.'s new book, *Eating Well for Optimal Health* and I decided to try adding Omega-3 fatty acids to my daily diet.
>
> "The result was so stunning I felt it to be my responsibility to write to tell you about it so that others might be helped. Each morning I grind up about two tablespoons of flax seeds in a spice grinder, which expanded to around 1/4 cup. After about two weeks of adding freshly ground flax seeds to my morning smoothie, yogurt or applesauce, my whole immune system strengthened so much that I was able even to eat candy.
>
> "I think it wasn't so much what I was eating in my prior diet or prepared foods, but what I wasn't eating. I think that's part of why the recommended natural diets help with yeast. There are more Omega-3 fatty acids included in them and less of the other lipids that either block the use of Omega-3s in the arachadonic acid synthesis pathway, or are toxic (like the trans fatty acids).
>
> "I wanted to let you know what worked for me. Thank you for your books and work you're doing trying to help others with candida."
>
> Sincerely,
> Cameron Thomas, M.S.
> Microbiology/Immunology

My Comments: Here are two important things for you to know.

+ You need Omega-3 fatty acids to enjoy good health.
+ Flax seeds are perhaps the best and most readily available source of Omega-3 fatty acids.

To obtain them go to your health food store and buy a bottle of flax seed oil (in a darkened bottle) from the refrigerator. Take 1–2 tbs. of flax seed oil a day. You can mix it with lemon juice and use it as a salad dressing, or you can take it straight. That's the way I take it each morning.

You can get the same essential nutrients from inexpensive, organically grown flax seeds. However you must first grind them in a food grinder and then store them in your freezer to keep them from becoming rancid. Then you can sprinkle a rounded tablespoon on your cereal, salad or soup once a day.

Professionals may also advise some of their patients to supplement their diets with evening primrose, borage, or black currant oils (Omega-6).

For more information about fats, I recommend the following books:

+ *Detoxification and Healing—The Key to Optimal Health,* Sidney M. Baker, M.D., Keats Publishing, 1997.
+ *Power Healing,* Leo Galland, M.D., Random House, 1998.
+ *Smart Fats,* Michael A. Schmidt, DC, Ltd., North Atlantic Books, P. O. Box 12327, Berkeley, CA 94712.
+ *Know Your Fats,* Mary Enig, Ph.D., Bethesdea Press, 2000.

REFERENCES

1. Baker, S.M., *Detoxification and Healing: The Key to Optimal Health,* Keats Publishing, New Canaan, CT, 1997, pp. 56–57.

2. Schmidt, M. *Smart Fats—How Dietary Fats and Oils Affect Mental, Physical and Emotional Intelligence,* Frog, Ltd., Berkeley, CA, 1997.

3. Smith, M.D., "The Stats of Fats", *Delicious!,* published by New Hope Natural Media, a division of Penton Media, May 1999.

4. Horrobin, D.F., Behan, P. O. and Behan, W.M.H., "Effect of high doses of essential fatty acids on the post-viral fatigue syndrome," *Acta. Neurol. Scand.,* 1990, 82:209–16.

5. Horrobin, D.F., "Essential Fatty Acids, Immunity and Viral Infections," *Journal of Nutritional Medicine,* 1990, pp. 145–151.

Magnesium

I f you're like most people you've been reading and hearing about the importance of calcium for many years. And many people, especially women, are taking calcium supplements in the hope of preventing osteoporosis and other disorders. Calcium is important, but so is magnesium.

During my pediatric residency and training many years ago, I used injections of magnesium sulfate to control elevated blood pressure in children with acute kidney disease. Magnesium was also used as a laxative. Yet, it wasn't until the mid-1960s, after reading several papers by Mildred Seelig that I began to learn about the importance of magnesium.

In the early 1980s I consulted Dr. Sidney M. Baker, former member of the clinical faculty of Yale University. I said, "Sid, tell me about magnesium." Here are part of his comments.

> "Magnesium deficiency is widespread. The average daily need for magnesium for an adult is between 500 mg and 1000 mg, and a lot of people simply aren't taking in that much. For my patients I recommend oral magnesium chloride."

Leo Galland, M.D.

A year or two later I learned more about magnesium from Dr. Galland, one of Dr. Baker's former associates. Like Baker, he pointed out that magnesium deficiency occurs much more often than is generally recognized. In discussing the food sources of magnesium he said,

> "The richest sources of magnesium are also the richest sources of essential fatty acids . . . Seed foods, including whole grains, nuts and beans. Other foods which are relatively rich

in magnesium include buckwheat, baking chocolate, cotton seed, tea, whole wheat and leafy green vegetables, including collard greens and parsley. The mineral is also plentiful in seafood, meats, nuts and fruit. What's more you can protect your magnesium stores by avoiding the magnesium wasters: saturated fats in soft drinks, especially those containing caffeine."

In his 1998 book, *Power Healing,* Galland said that Americans generally consume diets that are low in magnesium, which fail to meet the government's recommended daily allowance of 350 mg. He also said that people may become magnesium deficient even when their diets are adequate and that one of the reasons has to do with stress.

"The most exacting research on the stress/magnesium relationship has been done in Berlin and Paris using human volunteers. Men and women exposed to chronic noise, either traffic noise or occupational noise in a factory, develop irritability, fatigue and loss of concentration. . . Under conditions of mental or physical stress, magnesium is released from the cells and goes into the blood from which it is excreted into the urine. Chronic stress depletes the body of magnesium. The more stress to the individual, the greater the loss of magnesium . . .

"Administration of magnesium as a nutritional supplement raises blood levels of the mineral and buffers the response. Magnesium supplements can build resistance to the effects of stress . . . The best absorbed dietary supplement is magnesium glycinate, which is available in tablets, but there are many forms of magnesium available in drug stores and health food stores, and they may all be helpful to some people. "The dose needed varies from 100 mg to about 500 mg a day of elemental magnesium. . . Too much magnesium can cause diarrhea, which is its main and virtually its only side effect. Magnesium taken in quantities greater than 500 mg daily generally is very safe, except in people who suffer from kidney disease or are severely dehydrated."[1]

Melvyn Werbach, M.D.

In an article entitled "Nutritional Strategies for Treating Chronic Fatigue Syndrome," Melvyn R. Werbach, M.D., Assistant Clinical Professor at UCLA School of Medicine said,

> "A detailed review of the literature suggests a number of marginal nutritional deficiencies may have etiologic significance. These include deficiencies of various B vitamins, vitamin C, magnesium, sodium, zinc, L-tryptophan, L-carnitine, coenzyme Q10 and essential fatty acids."

In discussing magnesium Werbach reviewed a number of studies which have been published in the medical literature. Here are excerpts from his discussion.

> "Among patients seen in clinical settings, magnesium deficiency appears to be common . . . Although the literature is too sparse to draw firm conclusions, many CFS patients who have a magnesium deficiency could possibly derive benefit from magnesium supplementation."

Werbach then reviewed several clinical studies, including a placebo-controlled study. Those who received 100 mg. of magnesium intramuscularly for six weeks felt better compared to only 3 of 17 patients who received placebo. The red blood cell magnesium levels returned to normal in all of the patients who received magnesium, but in only one patient who received the placebo.

He also discussed the use of magnesium supplementation combined with malic acid. He reviewed a study by Drs. Guy Abraham and Jorge Flechas who carried out a study on their patients with fibromyalgia using magnesium combined with malic acid. The patients who were treated for an average of eight weeks with 200–600 mg of magnesium and 1200–2400 mg of malate daily showed a significant decrease in tender points. In commenting on their study he said,

> "While these results are promising, a subsequent double-blind crossover study of primary fibromyalgia patients who received 300 mg of magnesium and 1200 mg of malic acid or placebo in random order for four weeks, each with a two-week washout period in between, failed to find significant improvement in pain, tenderness and functional or psychological measures. . . If this study were to be repeated using twice the dosage lasting eight weeks, and including CFS patients, the results might be different."[2]

Alan Gaby, M.D.

This leader in the field of nutritional and preventive medicine, and author of the 1999 book *The Patient's Book of Natural Healing,* calls magnesium "the mineral that does it all." In discussing its therapeutic usage in his 1994 book, Gaby said it is important in helping people with fatigue, heart disease, asthma, depression, fibromyalgia, hypoglycemia, PMS and other disorders. And he said,

> "Because this nutrient is so critical in so many ways, and because supplementation is safe and inexpensive, I advise nearly all of my patients to take a magnesium supplement or a multivitamin and mineral formula that contains magnesium . . . It should be noted that many of the one tablet per day vitamin and mineral supplements contain very little magnesium."[3]

He also pointed out that too much magnesium may cause loose bowels in some people and that individuals with renal failure should not take magnesium without medical supervision.

Richard Firshein, D.O.

In an article entitled "Magnesium's Profound Effect on CFS," Dr. Firshein said,

". . . Magnesium allows our muscles to relax. If our bodies become calcium deficient we can borrow from a large reserve contained in our bones. But when our bodies become magnesium deficient, we must borrow from the already low supply in our muscles. . . As our muscles lose magnesium, calcium charges in to replace it, and as a result, our muscles grow tense and cramped. This can result in debilitating problems, especially exacerbation of chronic fatigue symptoms. Magnesium had a profound impact in the treatment of this disease."[4]

Firshein also told of his experiences in treating a number of his patients with a comprehensive program which included many therapeutic interventions. Treatment with magnesium was first on the list, using 500 mg of magnesium aspartate each day. He said,

"Magnesium alone, of course, can only do part of the job in a severe chronic illness. Other therapies were necessary."

Jacob Teitelbaum, M.D.

In discussing the multiple therapies required by the patient with CFS and fibromyalgia, Dr. Teitelbaum urges his patients to take a magnesium supplement. He said that this mineral is involved in hundreds of different body functions, but is routinely low in the American diet as a result of food processing.

"The average American diet supplies less than 300 mg of magnesium per day, while the average Asian diet supplies over 600 mg a day. I generally recommend taking malic acid, 800 mg and magnesium glycinate, 40 mg a day for eight months and then one-third this dose. If diarrhea and cramps are not a problem you can take up to twice this amount . . . If your magnesium is low your muscles will stay in spasm and your fibromyalgia will not resolve. This is one of the reasons that taking magnesium is so critical. . . In addition, magnesium is important for the muscles' and body's strength and energy."

In his continuing discussion Teitelbaum said that because more of your magnesium is inside the cells, magnesium blood tests are unreliable unless severe magnesium depletion occurs. He also said that if magnesium, which acts as a laxative, causes diarrhea the dosage can be cut back, then slowly increased "as is comfortable." If you have problems of any kind, you should discuss the dosage with your physician.

What magnesium preparation should you take? According to Teitelbaum,

> "Magnesium absorption is very difficult, which is why I like to use the glycinate forms. Therefore, the only forms I recommend are Fibrocare, the form in my From Fatigued to Fantastic Foundation Formula (both from *To Your Health*) or Pro Energy (from the *CFIDS Buyer's Club*). Plain magnesium oxide is also available and is the most inexpensive form of magnesium. Your body, however, may not absorb it well. If you choose to take magnesium oxide, take 500 milligrams per day."*

Martin Zucker

In an article entitled "5 Minerals That Can Save Your Heart" in the June 2000 issue of *Let's Live,* Zucker, a health writer, discussed magnesium, potassium, calcium, selenium and chromium. Based on the recommendations of Drs. Stephen Sinatra and Allan Magaziner, he listed magnesium first and included a delightful picture which illustrated the importance of magnesium. Here are excerpts of the article.

> "Whenever the subject of health arises in conversations I never hesitate to tout magnesium. I love magnesium. According to surveys, 75% of Americans are deficient and that can spell major trouble for your heart. . . Stress burns up magne-

---

*Adapted and excerpted from Dr. Teitelbaum's new book which will expand on the observations he made in his bestselling book, *From Fatigued to Fantastic*.

sium. If you don't have enough in your body your reactions to stress intensify.

"Chronic stress and magnesium deficiency can be deadly. That's because magnesium is involved in some 300 enzyme activities in the body. If it's depleted a lot can go wrong . . . I contacted two nutritionally oriented doctors who treat many heart patients, Stephen Sinatra, M.D., a cardiologist . . who is the author of *Heart Sense for Women* and Allan Magaziner, a specialist in nutritional and preventive medicine and author of *The Total Health Handbook*.

"'Magnesium is like King Arthur,' says Sinatra, 'all the other nutrients are the knights of the round table. People feel the benefit of supplementation rapidly. . .' Both Sinatra and Magaziner use magnesium along with other heart-friendly nutrients such as CoQ_{10} and vitamin E. The recommended dosage of magnesium is 400–800 mg daily."[5]

REFERENCES

1. Galland, L., *Power Healing,* Random House, 1998, pp 150–156.

2. Werbach, M.R., "Nutritional Strategies for Treating Chronic Fatigue Syndrome," Alternative Medicine Review, Vol. 5 No. 2, 20, pp 93–104.

3. Gaby, A., "Preventing and Reversing Osteoporosis," Prima Publishing, Rocklin, California, 95677, 1994, pp 39–45.

4. Firshein, R., www.immunesupport.com, 3-10-2000.

5. Zucker, M., "5 Minerals That Can Save Your Heart," *Let's Live,* June 2000.

Vitamin B₁₂

Although I rarely used vitamin B_{12} injections in treating my patients, over the years I've received anecdotal reports from professionals and nonprofessionals who said, "Vitamin B_{12} really helps." Here are excerpts from a letter I received from my patient, Linda, in the early 1990s.

> "I've been receiving vitamin B_{12} shots for several years to combat the allergic-tension-fatigue syndrome. When I take the shots I find I have much more energy and stamina to make it through a long day. The effects seem to wear off gradually within 8 to 10 days, so I try to get a shot once a week. The B_{12} shot is only one part of my health regimen, but when I miss a shot I definitely feel draggy. The shots may not work for everyone, but I certainly recommend them to my fellow sufferers."

Since Linda sent me that letter almost 10 years ago, she and her mother have continued to take weekly vitamin B_{12} shots. And in a recent conversation she said, "They really do help. When I miss a shot I can always tell a difference."

Comments by Charles Lapp, M.D.

In a three-page article entitled "Using Vitamin B_{12} for the Management of CFS" Charles Lapp, M.D., specialist in internal medicine and pediatrics and pioneer in treating CFIDS patients, told of the remarkable effectiveness of B_{12} injections in providing patients with increased energy levels, improved stamina and an enhanced sense of well-being. Here are excerpts from his article.

"In the late 1980s, Dr. Paul Cheney and I prepared several anecdotal reports of chronic fatigue syndrome (CFS) patients who improved when their primary care physicians administered B$_{12}$. This treatment was based on three articles that appeared in the New England Journal of Medicine, demonstrating that persons with CFS-like neurological symptoms and normal blood counts could benefit from the administration of Vitamin B$_{12}$ injections . . .

"Patients appeared to have a significant response at approximately 2000–2500 mcg. . . the effects lasted two to three days on average. However, many patients required up to six weeks to achieve regular consistent results . . . To obtain a continuous and satisfactory level of improvement, we now recommend injections of 3000 mcg. of cyanocobalamin every two to three days."

In his continuing discussion, Dr. Lapp said that two forms of B$_{12}$ are available to consumers: cyanocobalamin and hydroxycobalamin. He prefers the cyanocobalamin because it is less likely to cause adverse reactions and stings much less when injected. The cost of high-dose B$_{12}$ therapy is approximately $8–$10 per month.

"The patient can be taught to administer their own injection of B$_{12}$ using the same 1 cc insulin syringes diabetics use. They will need to obtain a supply of the B$_{12}$ solution from their physician. It comes in 10 ml. or 30 ml. multi-dose vials and should be stored in a dark place."

Dr. Lapp pointed out that patients taking large doses of Vitamin B$_{12}$ should supplement their diet with multivitamins containing B vitamins as well as folate.

In the concluding paragraph of his article, Lapp said,

"Persons with CFS who are interested in B_{12} therapy and are willing to take an injection two to three times a week should consult with their physician."

Observations by John V. Dommisse, M.D.

The more I've read and heard about the role of vitamin B_{12} in helping people with chronic fatigue, the more enthusiastic I've become about this simple, safe nutrient. In May 2000, Ken Gerdes, M.D., a Denver physician, sent me four pages of information from John Dommisse, M.D., an Arizona physician, (which was included in a syllabus in the March 2000 meeting of the American Academy of Environmental Medicine).

In his discussion, Dommisse said that, while most physicians know about the role of vitamin B_{12} in treating patients with pernicious anemia and related blood problems, they're often unaware of its role in helping people with mental symptoms. In his discussion he said,

> "This is unfortunate because the diagnosis of pernicious anemia is easily made and easily treated, whereas the B_{12}-deficient etiology of the affective disorder, the dementia, paranoid psychosis or violent behavior often remains unsuspected, undetected and therefore also untreated.
>
> "This is tragic because the deficiency can be fairly-easily reversed if diagnosed early enough and treated vigorously enough . . . This deficiency can be the cause of both bipolar and bipolar II disorders . . . Psychotic depression is particularly likely to be due to this deficiency. . .as shown by Levitt and Joffe.
>
> "*One other manifestation which appears to be emerging lately is fatigue.* Possibly first described by Ellis and Nasser* but also

---

*Ellis, F.R. and Nasser, S., "A pilot study of vitamin B_{12} in the treatment of tiredness." *British Journal of Nutrition*, 1973, April.

by Lindenbaum, et al.* Several of the author's patients who have been diagnosed as 'chronic fatigue syndrome' actually lost their tiredness when their hidden B$_{12}$ deficiency was corrected by criteria and methods described below. This seems to be the commonest cause of this syndrome and yet it is not even mentioned in the extensive literature that has recently been developed on the subject."

In his continuing discussion Dommisse said that blood levels are often used by physicians to determine vitamin B$_{12}$ deficiencies. And he said that the lab normal range is actually set too low and that "millions of patients with inadequate B$_{12}$ levels are passed as normal by the medical establishment, leaving them to be diagnosed as Alzheimer's (idiopathic) dementia and idiopathic depression, rather than being treated with the natural substance, that, if administered early and copiously enough, will cure their condition without any, or only minimal, side effects."

In discussing treatment he said,

> "There are two common misconceptions. (1) that most cases require intramuscular B$_{12}$; and (2) that an injection once a month or once every quarter is sufficient to counteract the neuropsychiatric effects of this deficiency in all or most cases."

He also said that almost all people with B$_{12}$ deficiency (except those with Crohn's Disease or terminal ileal resection) can be treated by vitamin B$_{12}$ orally in doses of 1000 to 5000 mg administered daily. And he said,

> "I personally decided, a long time ago, to maintain all my patients' serum levels above 1000 pg/ml, which is an optimal or ideal serum level. This substance is cheap and simple enough

---

*Lindenbaum, J., et al., "Neuropsychiatric Disorders Caused by Cobalamin Deficiency in the Absence of Anemia or Macrocytosis," *New Engl. J. Med.*, 318, 26:1720–8, 1988.

to take, especially orally, that neglecting to cover this base in one's practice should, in my opinion, be regarded as medical neglect."

Fifty-one references were cited by Dr. Dommisse. Here are a few of them:

McCallum, W.A.G., "Recoverable Psychiatric Illness, esp. Depression, Occurring with Low Serum Vitamin B_{12} Levels," J. Irish Med. Assoc., 1965: December: 187–92.

Solomon, J.G., "Remediable Causes of Dementia," Virginia Med, 1979, 106; 459–62.

Freidman, M.L., "B_{12}-deficit may be a common cause of dementia." Joint annual meeting of the American Geriatric Society and the American Federation for Aging. Research reported in Clinical Psychiatry News, 1988; 16, 9:10.

Warren, T., "Beating Alzheimer's," Garden City Park, NY, Avery Publishing Group, 1991.

Dommisse, J. V., "Subtle Vitamin B_{12} Deficiency and Psychiatry: An often unnoticed but devastating relationship?, Med. Hypoth., February 1991; 131–140.

Dommisse, J.V., "The Psychiatric Manifestations of B_{12} Deficiency," Primary Psyc., 1996, 3, 4(Apr), 18–21.

Dommisse, J.V., "The Experts Speak: The psychiatric manifestations of vitamin B deficiency," Clinical Pearls News, (I.T. Services), 3301 Alta Alden, #2, Sacramento, CA 95825 (1998).

Levitt, A.J. and Joffe, R.T., "Vitamin B_{12} Deficiency and Psychotic Depression," British Journal Psych., 1988; 153:266–267.

CoEnzyme Q_{10} (CoQ_{10})

first learned about this nutrient in 1987 from a book I found in a health food store entitled *The Miracle Nutrient, CoEnzyme Q_{10}* by Emile G. Blinzakov, M.D., and Gerald L. Hunt. I read the book from cover to cover and I was impressed. Here's a summary of some of the things I learned.

CoQ_{10} helps people with congestive heart failure and strengthens the immune system. It was first extracted from beef heart mitochondria in 1957. A great deal of work on this substance was carried out by Dr. Carol Folkers at the University of Texas, Austin. And on April 4, 1986, he received the Priestley Medal, the highest award bestowed by the American Chemical Society, in recognition of his work with CoQ_{10}, vitamin B_6 and B_{12}.

In spite of the studies by Dr. Folkers and other scientists, most members of the medical establishment ignored it until the 1990s. Then a few articles began to be published in the medical literature. Here's an excerpt from one of them.

> "A biochemical rationale for using CoQ_{10} in treating certain cardiovascular disease has been established. . . Its mechanism of action appears to be that of a free radical scavenger and/or direct membrane stabilizer."[1]

I've been so impressed with the beneficial effects of CoQ_{10} that I've taken it for the past decade and recommended it to my wife and three daughters as one of the nutrients that will strengthen their immune systems. I have also recommended it to my patients, including a 46-year-old Nashville woman who was troubled by fatigue, sinusitis, headache and recurrent attacks of asthma. On a comprehensive treatment program which included diet, nystatin, vitamin/minerals and CoQ_{10}, she improved remarkably. Here are excerpts from a letter she sent me.

"I'm enjoying better health than I can remember in my life. I'd never gone this long without a bronchial infection since I was 12 years old. I believe CoQ_{10} has contributed to my being able to stay well. . . Also, my mother and stepfather have been taking CoQ_{10} for over a year and have had no colds since they started taking it."

Several years ago in discussing their treatment recommendations for patients with chronic fatigue syndrome, Charles W. Lapp, M.D., and Paul R. Cheney, M.D., included the use of CoQ_{10}. Here's an excerpt from their recommendations.

"This enzyme . . . is thought to be involved in 95% of the cells metabolic reactions. It is particularly useful in improving fatigue, thought processes, muscular function and cardiac complaints. A threshold effect occurs and it may take five to six weeks for full benefit. We recommend 90 to 200 mg daily (one dose or divided) for a five to six weeks trial. . . We discontinue it if no benefit is noted in six weeks. We use the sublingual form to increase its bioavailability."[2]

In her 1997 book, *Miracle Cures,* Jean Carper includes a chapter on CoQ_{10}. Here are excerpts.

"CoQ_{10} is a unique antioxidant that reportedly penetrates the cells 'tiny energy factories' called mitochondria. Here oxygen is burned, giving cells energy to carry on the business of life. To efficiently burn energy, the mitochondria need CoQ_{10}. It is often called the 'spark' that starts and helps drive the mitochondria engines."[3]

Although most of Carper's discussion of this nutrient emphasizes the help it provides for people with heart problems, she also said that it is being tested in patients with degenerative neurological diseases at major medical centers, including the University of Rochester Medical School and the University of California, San Diego.

In an article in _Nutrition Science News,_ Carmia Borek, Ph.D., research professor, Tufts University School of Medicine, discussed the many benefits of CoQ$_{10}$ in which she said CoQ$_{10}$ is essential for energy generation and antioxidant protection. It is present in all foods we eat. Rich dietary sources include almonds, ocean salmon, sardines, spinach and meat—especially organs and muscles that contain high levels of mitochondria, such as heart and other muscles.[4]

In a four-page discussion entitled "Cancer, the Next Frontier," Carper cited Danish researcher Knut Lockwood, whose patient with metastatic cancer went into complete remission. The treatment program for this patient included large doses (300 mg per day) of CoQ$_{10}$, plus other nutrients, including vitamin C, E, selenium and Omega-3 fatty acids.

If you'd like to learn more about CoQ$_{10}$, get a copy of the 176-page book by Stephen Sinatra, M.D., a Fellow of the American College of Cardiology, entitled _The Coenzyme Q$_{10}$ Phenomenon._ He said that in spite of the importance of CoQ$_{10}$, most American physicians either don't know about it or ignore the possibility that it can help their patients. Here are excerpts from Dr. Sinatra's book.

> "Think of the body as a fine-tuned car. Functioning on low levels of CoQ$_{10}$ would be similar to running a car on a low-octane fuel. With such poor octane energy fuel, the cylinders in the car's high-performance engine (where the gasoline is ignited) would not have sufficient force to move the pistons evenly. Energy that then drives the car would be inadequate, resulting in misfiring pistons and sluggish undependable movement. Similarly, _the human body must have high octane fuel_

to create the energy to carry on the basic processes of life . . ." (emphasis added)

In the final chapter of this book, Dr. Sinatra, in discussing the future of CoQ_{10}, said,

> "Although rationale for treatment of a wide variety of diseases has been published in a number of controlled and uncontrolled studies, it continues to be underutilized by most American physicians . . . When a substance like Coenzyme Q_{10} is touted for so many pathological ailments it sounds just too good to be true. This probably raises much skepticism and rightly so. . . *Coenzyme Q_{10} is a proven nutrient with prophylactic and therapeutic value. When taken in combination with a healthy diet and proper supplementation CoQ_{10} has a greater chance for achieving maximum potential."*[5] (emphasis added)

How much CoQ_{10} should you take? What supplements are best? Based on research studies carried out and cited by Sinatra, all of the CoQ_{10} supplements available commercially are not "equally bioavailable." In discussing the various products, he said that most CoQ_{10} is made in Japan and sold to various companies but the packagings and preparations differ. He also pointed out that new research shows that CoQ_{10} in soft-gel capsules, which are both water- and fat-soluble, are superior to the dry form because more CoQ_{10} gets into the bloodstream.

When people ask, "How much CoQ_{10} should I take?" I usually say, "Based on information I've read in articles and books, I'd recommend at least 100 mg a day if you're 'sick and tired.' And if you have more serious problems, including heart disease or cancer, I'd take 400 mg or more. *Take as much as you can afford!"*

If you'd like a comprehensive discussion of CoQ_{10} and its benefits, I urge you to get a copy of the 1998 book by Stephen T. Sinatra, M.D., a Connecticut board-certified specialist who has treated thousands of patients with CoQ_{10} supplementation over the past decade. Here are excerpts from the back cover of his book.

"Hundreds of scientific studies and thousands of clinical applications have shown that Co-Enzyme Q_{10} may be one of the greatest 20th-century medical advances for the treatment of a wide variety of cardiovascular disorders from angina and arrhythmias to congestive heart failure in hypertension. . . Despite the large body of clinical evidence, Co-Q_{10} is either unknown or ignored by most physicians."

Although Dr. Sinatra focuses especially on its use in patients with heart problems, he said that it has applications for many other disorders, including cancer, periodontal disease, diabetes, energy and stamina.

My Comments: Although CoQ_{10} won't solve all of your health problems, it's an important member of the "team" which will enable you to conquer your fatigue. You'll also need to do the things I've discussed elsewhere in this book, including: consume nutritious foods, avoid chemical pollutants in your home and office and take prescription and nonprescription anti-yeast medications to control the yeast overgrowth in your digestive tract.

REFERENCES

1. Frishman, W.H., "CoEnzyme Q_{10}—A new drug for cardiovascular disease," *Journal of Clinical Pharmacology,* 1990; 30(7):596–608.

2. Lapp, C.W. and Cheney, P.R.. Personal communication.

3. Carper, J., *Miracle Cures,* Harper Collins Publishing, New York, NY, 1997.

4. Borek, C., *Nutrition Science News,* July 1999.

5. Sinatra, S.T., *The Coenzyme Q_{10} Phenomenon,* Keats, NTC/Contemporary Publishing Group, Chicago, IL, 1998, pp. 24, 28–29.

Hypothyroidism

According to a leaflet I received from the Thyroid Foundation of America, Inc.,

"Some patients with mild hypothyroidism may not show any symptoms. Yet, such patients may note improvement in their sense of well-being after being treated with thyroid hormone.

"With more severe hypothyroidism you may begin to feel run down, slow, depressed, sluggish, cold, tired and may lose interest in normal daily activities. Other symptoms may include dryness and brittleness of hair, dry and itchy skin, constipation, muscle cramps and increased menstrual flow in women."[*]

I became interested in hypothyroidism during my early years of pediatric practice because of my experience with a child who was sluggish and who did not develop normally until he was put on supplemental thyroid. In reading the medical literature I was especially impressed by the observations of Broda O. Barnes, M.D., who began publishing articles in the peer-reviewed literature in the 1940s. Then in 1976 Barnes published a book, *Hypothyroidism, The Unsuspected Illness*.[†]

He recommended basal temperature tests in determining a thyroid deficiency. According to his original instructions, people were asked to use an ordinary thermometer, put it in an armpit

---

[*]Thyroid Foundation of America, Inc., Ruth Sleeper Hall, RSL 350, 40 Parkman Ave., Boston, MA 02114–2698.
[†]Barnes, B.O., with Dalton, L., *Hypothyroidism, The Unsuspected Illness*, Harper and Row, New York, 1976.

and leave it for *10* minutes. If the thermometer readings were subnormal, hypothyroidism appeared to be a definite possibility.

During the past decade several physicians I've consulted have reported the basal temperature under the tongue for five minutes worked just as well. In 1994 Dr. Ken Gerdes, a Denver physician who had used the under-the-tongue method, said,

> "If a patient's temperature is consistently under 97.4 or 97.6 in the morning I prescribe thyroid supplements, including Armour thyroid tablets (which contains T4 and T3) and additional T3."

In January 2000 I called Dr. Gerdes to get an update on his recommendations. Here are excerpts from our conversation.

> "In my experience, many people, especially women, who are deficient in thyroid may be helped by thyroid supplementation. . . As you know, there are several different types of these products. . . Many patients improve by simply giving enough thyroid to move the TSH into the active end of the normal range. *Relying on temperature alone seems hazardous as there seem to be non-thyroid factors which influence the temperature.*
>
> "Recently the availability of testing for "free T3" and "free T4" allows us to normalize each of these variables, which may provide even more appropriate thyroid treatment than we have by moving the TSH into the active range.
>
> "I've already found several patients with an active end of the 'normal' range TSH who are distinctly low in free T3. When this information about 'free T3' and 'free T4' gets spread widely, it might just make the TSH obsolete. . . There are plenty of miserable people on thyroid at 'normal' levels."

Then in April 2000, Dr. Gerdes sent me a four-page discussion entitled "A Radical New Approach to Hypothyroidism" which had been presented by Dr. John V. Dommisse at the March 2000 conference of the American Academy of Environmental

Medicine. In his exciting presentation, Dr. Dommisse said that during the past 11 years he had treated hundreds of hypothyroid patients with a combination of Levothyroid, Synthroid (T4) and Armour thyroid or Levoxyl (which contains T4 and T3) and Cytomel (which is pure T3). And he said,

> "I'm gratified to report that the prestigious *New England Journal of Medicine* (NEJM, by Dr. R. Bunevicius and colleagues) has finally . . . published a paper showing that many hypothyroid patients function significantly better when 50 mcg of their previous T4-only treatment is substituted with 12.5 mcg of T3."*

Dommisse also pointed out that a number of publications over the past 15 years have documented the greater efficacy of T4 plus T3 as compared to T4-only in treating people with hypothyroidism. In his discussion he pointed out that until recently physicians who were prescribing T3 were often "thought by their colleagues to be practicing on the fringes of medicine."

He cited an editorial by Dr. Anthony Toft, in the same issue of NEJM as the Bunevicius report, which stated that T3 in treating hypothyroidism is "vital for optimal thyroid function." In his continuing discussion, Dr. Dommisse said,

> "No matter how certain one may be that one's approach is the correct one, it is still very hard to 'paddle against the stream'—especially when the stream consists of the considered opinion of all of the top endocrinologists in the U.S. . .
> "The latest development in the loosening of the stranglehold that T4-only treatment has on hypothyroid patients has come in the form of a book written by an associate professor

---

*Bunevicius, R., et al., "Effects of thyroxine as compared with thyroxine-plus-triiodothyronine in patients with hypothyroidism," *New England Journal of Medicine*, 1999; 340:424–9.

of endocrinology at Baylor Medical College—and published by Ballantine Books in June 1999."*

In discussing this book, Dr. Dommisse said that the author, Dr. Ridha Arem, is convinced that some patients with "normal" thyroid blood values are actually hypothyroid and he puts them on a therapeutic trial of thyroid hormone treatment.

> "He makes the further observations that some patients on T4-only treatment do not do well enough and are not returned to their pre-hypothyroid state, and he adds Cytomel, 5–10 mcg, two to three times daily. All of them have improved and have been restored to their normal level of functioning."

_____

*Arem, R., *The Thyroid Solution: A Mind-Body Program for Beating Depression and Regaining Your Emotional and Physical Health*, New York: Ballantine Books, June 1999.

Exercise

n discussing the importance of regular exercise in their wonderful *Encyclopedia of Natural Medicine,* Michael T. Murray, N.D., and Joseph E. Pizzorno, N.D. said,

> "Regular physical exercise is obviously a major key to good health. We all know this, yet only a small fraction (fewer than 20%) of Americans exercise on a regular basis. . . Exercise is absolutely vital. . . The entire body benefits from regular exercise, largely as a result of improved cardiovascular and respiratory function. Simply stated, exercise enhances the transport of oxygen and nutrients into cells.
>
> "At the same time exercise enhances the transport of carbon dioxide and waste products from the tissues of the body to the bloodstream and ultimately to the eliminative organs. As a result, regular exercise increases stamina and energy levels."[1]

These benefits seem obvious to physicians and the public today, but it wasn't always this way. A little over 60 years ago my sister Nancy (as was the custom in those days) was kept in bed for a week following an appendix operation. Her inactivity led to a blood clot in her leg. Other patients following operations have developed similar complications. By contrast, today hospitalized patients following major surgery procedures, including open heart surgery, get out of bed and begin walking in 24 hours (or less) following surgery.

Here's another example: mothers, following the birth of a baby, were kept in bed for a week or more. Then doctors gradually realized that this period of inactivity led to problems of various sorts, including weakness, fatigue and postpartum depression.

In an article entitled "Exercise: Practical Treatment for the Patient with Depression and Chronic Fatigue," Dr. Charles W. Smith recommended exercises of many types, including walking, dancing, swimming and bicycling.[2]

And obstetrician/gynecologist Dr. Joe F. McIlhaney, Jr., said,

> "There are several direct rewards for anyone who starts a regular program of exercise . . . *When patients complain to me of feeling tired or not having much energy, I assure them that if they will begin exercising, within two weeks they will feel like different people.*"[3] (emphasis added)

How You Can Enjoy Exercising

You may say, "Exercise is boring and it isn't much fun." I understand what you're saying and I feel the same way; especially if you're exercising by yourself. You'll enjoy exercising if you walk with a friend, play a game of any kind or join a class. Both the exercise and the companionship will help you overcome your feelings of fatigue.

Georgia Deaton, who has worked with me for over 40 years, became tired and depressed after open heart surgery and the subsequent death of her husband. Now she's back on the job, working part-time and doing a superb job. To keep physically fit and mentally alert, she joins others in a one-hour cardiac rehab class three times a week.

Comments by Jacob Teitelbaum, M.D.

This young physician is an *authority* in treating patients with chronic fatigue. Here are four reasons why he's an authority.

1. He developed CFS soon after medical school and it took him many months to recover.

125

2. He's a board-certified internist with impeccable personal and professional credentials.

3. He recently carried out a placebo-controlled, scientific study using the antifungal drug Sporanox on patients with fibromyalgia (see www.endfatigue.com).

4. He's the author of the popular book *From Fatigued to Fantastic* and he emphasizes the importance of multiple therapeutic interventions, including antifungal drugs.

In discussing exercise, Teitelbaum said,

"Exercise is very important for your sense of well-being. Fibromyalgia patients often find that when they exercise they feel exhausted the next day. . . Wait until you're 8–10 weeks into treatment and feeling better, then . . . as your health starts to improve, slowly add exercise to your regime. Begin with something gentle, such as walking or swimming. . . Soon, you will find your ability and stamina are normalizing. Give yourself time to slowly build up . . . Increasing your daily walk by 3–5 minutes each week as is comfortable.

"I recommend walking as the primary exercise during the initial stages of recovery. Walking conditions the heart and muscles and is easy on the joints and ligaments. When you walk outdoors, you can also enjoy the fresh air. . . Fresh air is good for the lungs and clears the mind . . . When the weather is chilly, walk around your local mall."[4]

Suggestions from the *Harvard Women's Health Watch*

According to an article in the June 2000 issue of this publication,

"Nearly 17 million women went day hiking at least once in 1998. . . Outdoor hiking offers many of the same benefits as walking; a reduced risk of heart disease and diabetes, stronger bones and improved mood. It's also a great calorie burner."

Beginning hikers who have led sedentary lives were urged to prepare themselves physically for the trail. But before hiking or starting on any new exercise venture, readers should go to their physician for a consultation. And before taking a hike, stretching is vital.

The article recommended two kinds of stretch: Achilles tendon stretch and back stretch. In the Achilles tendon stretch you stand upright, arms length from a wall. Then you place your left leg forward with knee bent while keeping your right leg and back straight. Then lean slowly forward to the waist. Other instructions in the article include purchasing good footwear and a ski or trekking pole to help you keep your balance, especially if you're wearing a backpack.

Single copies of this issue of *Harvard Women's Health Watch* are available for $5 each. Write or e-mail Harvard Health Publications, P.O. Box 421073, Palm Coast, FL 32142-1073 or harvardpro@palmcoastd.com.

REFERENCES

1. Murray, M.T. and Pizzorno, J.E., *Encyclopedia of Natural Medicine,* Revised Second Edition, Prima Publishing, p. 35, 1998.

2. Smith, C.W., Jr., "Exercise: Practical Treatment with Depression and Chronic Fatigue," *Primary Care,* 1991, 18(2):271–81.

3. McIlhaney, J.F. with Nethery, S., *1250 Health Questions Women Ask,* Baker Book House Company, Grand Rapids, MI and Focus on the Family Publishing, Colorado Springs, CO 1992, p. 816.

4. Teitelbaum, J., *From Fatigued to Fantastic,* Avery Publishing Company, 1996, pp. 72–73.

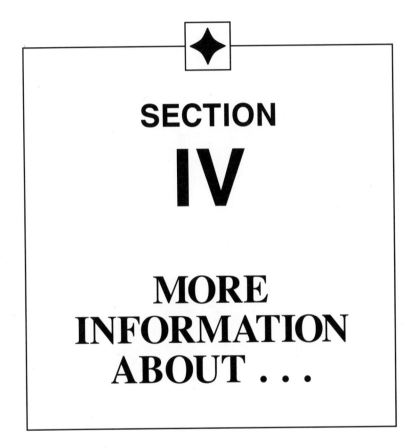

SECTION

IV

MORE
INFORMATION
ABOUT . . .

Diet

I f you're confused about the foods you should eat and those you should avoid, you have a lot of company. Here are some of the reasons.

Thousands of articles about nutrition and diet have been published in both the medical and lay press during the 1980s and 1990s. During these same years, hundreds of books have been written and published by professional and lay writers providing you with recommendations.

On the one hand you were told that you'll enjoy good health if you stop eating eggs, pork chops and steaks because they're "bad for you." So you were encouraged to eat less fat and the food producers responded by producing foods that were low in fat or "fat free." Many people ate fewer animal products and obtained their calories from other sources, including candy, colas, crackers, cookies and other snack foods which contained partially hydrogenated fats. They also ate more bagels, bread, spaghetti and pizza. I read that fast food eateries were selling more pizza than hamburgers. And in the 1990s more and more Americans of all ages (including children) became overweight—even obese.

Then the reaction set in. Books and articles were written which sold millions of copies, including books by Barry Sears and his "zone diets," Morrison Bethea and his book *Sugar Busters!* Last but not least are Robert Atkins' books which have sold millions of copies. In an interview with Dr. Atkins published in the February 2000 issue of *Let's Live,* Beth Salmon said,

> "Everywhere from the morning news to late night talk shows, Robert Atkins, M.D., has been debated, criticized and on occasion condemned. But despite the controversy, the

American public still buys his books by the truckload, crediting his diet with not only helping them to shed pounds, but also with saving their lives. . . For those readers who may not know, briefly tell us what the Atkins diet is."

In responding, Dr. Atkins said,

> "It's a life-long nutritional philosophy, focusing on the consumption of nutrient-dense, unprocessed foods and nutrient supplementation. It restricts processed and refined carbohydrates such as high sugar foods, breads, pastas and cereals. The maintenance level of the diet allows a complete choice of proteins, fats, legumes and vegetables, as well as unrefined whole grains."[1]

In his continuing discussion, Atkins said that he had been following a maintenance diet which he's been off and on for 36 years and that he probably eats 50 servings of vegetables a week. He said, "It's basically a protein and vegetables diet."

Those who disagree with Sears, Bethea and Atkins include Drs. Dean Ornish, Andrew Weil, John McDougall and followers of the late Nathan Pritikin. (After meeting Pritikin at a conference in the early 1970s, I became one of his fans and served as a consultant for his Longevity Research Institute.) In my book *The Yeast Connection and the Woman* I cited the observations of Pritikin, Ornish and McDougall. And I said,

> "Evidence is piling up at a fast pace, confirming that fruits and vegetables are full of exotic health-promoting compounds that boost bodily defenses against disease in all sorts of ways. There's no doubt about it. The message is clear. *Vegetarians, and even meat eaters who eat a lot of plant foods, enjoy impressive health advantages.*"

In a special feature article in the May 2000 *Nutrition Action Healthletter,* "DIET vs. DIET—Battle of the Bulge Doctors,"

Bonnie Liebman reviewed the "Great Nutrition Debate" held by the U.S. Department of Agriculture in February 2000. In her discussion she said,

> "It should have been called a 'Great Dieting Debate. . .' Sparks flew between Drs. Robert Atkins, Barry Sears, Dean Ornish, John McDougall, Morrison Bethea and other panelists. *What didn't fly was good research."*

Liebman quoted Susan Roberts, head of the Energy Metabolism Laboratory at the Jean Mayer U.S. Department of Agriculture Human Nutrition Research Center on Aging at Tufts University in Boston, who said,

> "I'm not aware of a single trustworthy piece of evidence that suggests that high protein diets like Atkins' are a healthy way to eat. . . The epidemiological studies point to fruits, vegetables and whole grains as health foods."

Elsewhere in the article Liebman gave rules for healthy weight loss which included these comments,

> "Until better diet studies are done, our advice is to exercise and make sure your diet is healthy. It should be:
>
> ✦ low in saturated and transfat to cut your risk of heart disease and possible colon and prostate cancer
> ✦ rich in vegetables and fruits to cut your risk of cancer, heart disease and stroke
> ✦ low in 'largely' empty calorie foods."[2]*

Here's a question many people have been and are asking: "Would we be healthy if we all became vegetarians?" Answers to this question also stir up controversy. Since I first met Pritikin

---

*You can obtain additional information from www.cspinet.org.

I've eaten less meat and eggs and more vegetables, fruits and whole grains. Yet, I've received information from authoritative sources which showed that for many centuries people who ate a varied diet, *which included beef, pork, chicken and other animal foods,* enjoyed good health. They also developed less heart (and other vascular) trouble and cancer—diseases which kill so many Americans today.

David Rowland, author of a Canadian health magazine, in an editorial published a couple of years ago said in effect, "If our Canadian ancestors in the 18th and 19th Century had been vegetarians, they would not have survived because vegetables don't thrive under the snow."

In a comprehensive (and somewhat hostile) discussion of vegetarianism in the July 2000 issue of the *Townsend Letter for Doctors and Patients*, Steven Byrnes, N.D., discussed many "myths" about the supposed benefits of becoming a vegetarian. He also cited references to cookbooks and other data from the 1800s which showed that people eating varied diets, including animal foods, were healthy and lived long lives. In his discussion he pointed out that many of the health problems people face today are caused by

> ". . . *consumption of margarine and other transfatty acids, lifeless packaged 'foods,' processed vegetable oils, pasteurized/homogenized milk, commercially raised livestock and plant foods and refined sugar. These are the real culprits in our modern epidemics of cancer and coronary heart disease and other chronic illnesses.*" (emphasis added)[3]

Byrnes also cited the observations of Dr. Weston Price, who went around the world in the 1920s and 1930s photographing elderly native peoples who ate food from many sources, including animals. About 25 years ago I read Dr. Price's book *Nutrition* *and Physical Degeneration* which was first published over 60 years ago.*

In this book, Price showed pictures of healthy people eating native diversified diets which included animal products. By contrast, those consuming Western diets loaded with sugars, starches and processed fats were troubled by health problems of many types.

Soy Foods—a Controversial Subject

In the June 2000 issue of *Consumers' Research*† magazine entitled "Limited Health Claims for Soy Products," John Hinkle‡ said,

> "Vegetarians and health enthusiasts have known for years that foods rich in soy protein offer a good alternative to meat, poultry and other animal-based products. As consumers have pursued healthy lifestyles in recent years, consumption of soy foods has risen steadily. . . Last October the Food and Drug Administration gave food manufacturers permission to put labels on products high in soy protein indicating that these foods may help lower heart-disease risk."[4]

In his continuing discussion Hinkle said that no sooner than the FDA proposed the health claim regulation, critics began to question the safety of certain soy products, including *isoflavones* or *phytoestrogens* (a weak form of estrogen.) He quoted a number of authorities, including Margo Woods, D.Sc., Associate Profes-

---

*This book is available today from the Price-Pottenger Nutrition Foundation, 1-800-366-3748. E-mail: info@pricepottenger.org. See also reference to this foundation in Section V.

†For a copy of this article, send a stamped, self-addressed envelope and $5 to For a copy of this newsletter, send a mailing label and $5 *Consumers' Research* magazine which is published monthly by Consumers' Research, Inc., 800 Maryland Ave., N.E., Washington, DC 20002.

‡Mr. Hinkle is a member of FDA's Public Affairs staff, and writes for FDA Consumer, from which the Consumer Research article was excerpted.

sor of Medicine at Tufts University, who has studied soy's effects in postmenopausal women, who said, "There's a lot of emerging data and it's confusing. In the meantime we should be cautious." She said her concerns are centered mainly on isoflavone supplements and she's "much more comfortable recommending soy as a whole food . . . It's just too big a leap to assume that a pill could do the same thing."

In a companion *Consumers' Research* article, "What You Also Need to Know About Soy," Beatrice Trum Hunter* said,

> "Despite many alleged benefits of soy which are being promoted enthusiastically, there's also a downside, which is largely being ignored. Soy contains many anti-nutrients. Only one is mentioned briefly in the FDA article."

Hunter listed a number of anti-nutrients, including phytic acid, which may prevent the absorption of some minerals and hemaglutinins—substances that may make red blood cells clump together. She said that many of these anti-nutrients present in soybeans can be reduced by proper heat treatment or by sprouting the beans.

> "The only satisfactory method known to deactivate these anti-nutrients is by means of fermentation . . . The main fermented soybean products are tempeh (a soybean-based entree), miso (a soybean paste used in soup and sauces) and natto (fermented whole soybeans). . . Soybean products such as tofu and bean curd, familiar and available to Americans, are *not* fermented."[5]

---

*Beatrice Trum Hunter is Food Editor at *Consumers' Research* and author of a number of books concerning food topics of importance to consumers. Her most recent ones include *The Great Nutrition Robbery, The Mirage of Safety* and *The Sugar Trap and How to Avoid It.* You may send your questions about food to Beatrice Trum Hunter, c/o Consumers' Research, 800 Maryland Ave. N.E., Washington, D.C. 20002. For a personal reply enclose a self-addressed stamped envelope.

Other "downsides" of soy products cited by Hunter include the frequent partial hydrogenation of soy oil and anti-thyroid properties. She also said, "At present, soy is among the *major* food allergens in the American diet."

In another article in the July 2000 *Townsend Letter,* Sally Fallon* and Mary G. Enig, Ph.D.,† discussed the intensive current marketing of soybeans during the decade of the 1990s. They said,

> "The push for more soy has been relentless and global in its reach. Soy protein is now found in most supermarket breads . . . Soy is now sold to the upscale customer . . . as a miracle substance that will help prevent heart disease and cancer, whisk away hot flashes, build strong bones and keep us forever young."

In their continuing discussion they pointed out the "dark side" of consuming too many soybean products. They said that studies by a number of researchers indicate that one of the highly publicized soy ingredients, *isoflavones,* are toxic. This soy derivative may cause problems in various ways, including enzyme inhibitors, endocrine disruption, reproductive problems and increased allergic reactions.

> "For most of us giving up steak and eating veggie burgers instead will not bring blood cholesterol levels down. . . Studies in which cholesterol levels were lowered either through diet or drugs have consistently resulted in a greater number of deaths in the treatment groups than in controls . . . Deaths from cholesterol lowering measures in the U.S. have fueled a

---

*Sally Fallon is the author of *Nourishing Challenges: The Cookbook that Challenges Politically Correct Nutrition and the Diet Dictocrats,* Second edition, 1999, New Tens Publishing, 877-707-1776 or 219-268-2601.

†Mary G. Enig, Ph.D., is the author of *Know Your Fats: The Complete Primer for Understanding the Nutrition of Fats, Oils and Cholesterol,* 2000, www.bethesda press.com.

60-billion-dollar-a-year cholesterol-lowering industry, but have not saved us from the ravages of heart disease."[6]

Carbohydrates—Another Controversy

Complex carbohydrates, especially vegetables and fruits, are good for you. No one questions their value in providing important nutrients of many types, including vitamins, minerals and phytopharmaceuticals with complicated names. They're especially beneficial if you consume a wide variety, provided they aren't loaded with pesticides or other toxic chemicals.

Whole grains are also nutritious and are "good" carbohydrates if you aren't allergic or sensitive to them. Wheat, especially, causes adverse reactions in many people. So does corn, especially if it's refined. But grain alternatives, including amaranth and quinoa, may be tolerated by wheat-sensitive people.

Sugars derived from cane, beet or corn are "bad" carbohydrates. Here are several reasons.

1. They've been stripped of minerals, vitamins and other nutrients. According to a USDA report, "Sugars and Sweeteners," the average American is consuming an estimated 154+ pounds of caloric sugars each year. In so doing the calories obtained replace those that could and should be obtained from the good carbohydrates.

2. Digestion of these simple sugars stimulates insulin release from the pancreas. Insulin lowers the blood sugar and makes people irritable, hungry or jittery and causes them to crave and eat more sweets. One of the results is that more Americans are becoming obese.

3. Last, but not least, simple sugars encourage multiplication of the yeast *Candida albicans* in the digestive tract. A research study in the early 1990s at St. Jude Hospital in Memphis, showed that mice receiving dextrose in their

diet (as compared to controls) had a 200-fold increase in *Candida albicans* proliferation.

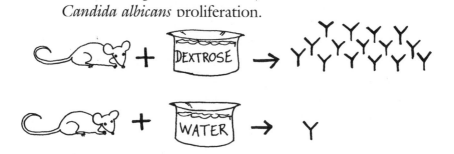

Recently, I received new information about carbohydrates from my friend Beatrice Trum Hunter, a writer on food issues. She sent me an article from the May 2000 issue of *Prepared Foods* entitled "Cutting Edge Carbohydrates" by Alphons G.J. Voragen, Department of Food Technology and Nutritional Sciences, Wageningen Agricultural University, The Netherlands.* Here are excerpts.

"A number of normal dietary carbohydrates also have the ability to function as prebiotics or fat replacers. Prized for their ability to enhance the nutritional profile of foods, they include nondigestible oliogosaccharides (NDOs), resistant starches and carbohydrate-based fat replacers.

". . . NDOs such as inulin are increasingly being added to foods, particularly in some European countries and Japan. NDOs function as prebiotics because they are neither hydrolyzed nor absorbed in the upper part of the gastrointestinal tract. As a result, they selectively stimulate the growth and/or activity of one or a limited number of 'healthy' bacterial species resident in the colon."

In the concluding paragraphs of his article, the author said,

_____
*Can be reached by phone at 31317-483209. Fax: 313317-484893. E-mail: <u>fons.vor agen@chem.fdsci.wau.nl</u>.

"Despite the abundant research done on the beneficial effects of carbohydrates, there is still much to learn. . . Improvement in our understanding of the role of carbohydrates in normal cell processes and disease is likely to lead to the development of new dietary oligosaccharide products for the prevention or treatment of pathogen colonizations of the gastrointestinal tract. With this larger knowledge, we will be able to tailor-make novel dietary carbohydrates."

My Comments: If you'd like more information about diets, read the *Nutrition Action Healthletter, Consumers' Research,* the *PPNF Newsletter* and other publications I've listed on pages 364–365. Here's a summary of the advice I give to my patients, family members and my friends.

+ *Fruits and vegetables are good for you.* You should consume at least 7–10 portions a day. If possible purchase organically-grown foods. If such foods are unavailable, buy produce from local growers who do *not* overload them with pesticides.
+ *Keep your intake of sugar and other simple carbohydrates to a minimum.* I read that in George Washington's day the average American consumed six pounds of sugar a year. It was used as a condiment. By contrast, today the average American consumes 140—160 pounds of cane sugar, beet sugar and corn sugar—much of the latter is in the form of high fructose corn syrup.
+ *Eat good fats, including nuts every day.* They are a superb snack food. (See also pages 277–280) Also take a tablespoon of flax seed oil every day or grind up flax seeds and sprinkle a tablespoon or two on salad. Use olive oil in cooking. You can also use it as a spread in place of butter.
+ *Avoid bad fats,* especially the hydrogenated and partially hydrogenated fats which you'll find in many, many foods

on the shelves of your grocery store, including crackers and cakes. They're put there especially to make the shelf-life longer. Also avoid the high-fat meats, including "hot dogs," hamburgers, bacon and luncheon meats. Trim off fat from beef, pork, chicken or lamb.

✦ *Vary your diet. Don't eat the same foods every day.* Eat some animal foods but you don't need to include them in every meal, or even every day. (I haven't forgotten all of the information I received from Nathan Pritikin and his followers.)

✦ *Include whole eggs in your diet several times a week—or even every day.* Mary Enig, Ph.D., (and others) says that the experts who have advised you to avoid eggs and other cholesterol-containing foods are wrong. Eggs are loaded with nutrients and a lot better for you than Egg Beaters(TM). But cook your eggs well to make sure you kill the salmonella bacteria.

✦ *Butter is okay—not too much or too often.* It's a lot better than hydrogenated fats found in margarines.

✦ *Eat seafood two or three times a week—especially fish caught offshore.* But don't eat the same fish every day if it comes from a river, lake or pond. Such fish may be contaminated with mercury, pesticides or other chemicals.

✦ *Take "insurance" vitamin/mineral/antioxidants every day.*

REFERENCES

1. Salmon, B., *Let's Live,* February 2000.

2. Liebman, B., *Nutrition Action Healthletter,* "DIET vs. DIET," May 2000.

3. Byrnes, S., *Townsend Letter for Doctors and Patients,* 911 Tyler St., Port Townsend, WA 98368-6581. www.tldp.com. E-mail: tldp@olympus.net., July 2000.

4. Hinkle, J., *Consumers' Research,* "Limited Health Claims for Soy Products," June 2000.

5. Hunter, B.T., *Consumers' Research,* "What You Also Need to Know About Soy," June 2000.

6. Fallon, S., Enig, M., *Townsend Letter for Doctors and Patients,* 911 Tyler St., Port Townsend, WA 98368-6581. www.tldp.com. E-mail: tldp@olympus.net., July 2000.

Chemicals

During my childhood in the 1920s, my parents, siblings and I lived on a 3-acre "mini" farm, along with one or two cows and 100 chickens. Scattered over our home-place were many oak trees and my mother enjoyed growing vegetables and flowers. Compost piles made from decaying leaves and cow manure provided nutrients for these plants. My mother grew so many vegetables that I earned pocket money by selling them to the neighbors.

Neighbors and friends would say, "Mrs. Crook has a green thumb. Her vegetables grow better than anybody else's." I can't recall my mother spraying insecticides, weed killers or other chemicals in our garden.

I walked to school a mile away, I skated, rode my pony or my bicycle after school and during the summer. I played tennis, baseball and other sports. (We had a tennis court and a small baseball "diamond" on our back lot.) In addition, I had to do chores like cutting the grass and raking leaves, so I spent a lot of time outdoors.

Few automobiles came down the road to pollute the air with lead and other toxic substances contained in automobile exhaust. Houses were made out of wood or brick and heated by radiators and wood fires. Clothing and home furnishings were made from natural fabrics which didn't put out offensive odors. When I was growing up, we ate good food and breathed clean air.

I don't want life to sound perfect, because it wasn't. Family members and friends and neighbors experienced health problems almost unheard of today. One of my sisters almost died with typhoid fever and a brother almost died with pneumonia. Scarlet fever, measles and other childhood diseases caused death and disability in many people. So did diphtheria, "lock jaw" (tetanus) and polio.

During the past 70 years amazing, fantastic and breathtaking changes have taken place. Because of advances in medicine many lives have been saved and much suffering has been prevented or relieved. Although I don't want to go back to the "good old days," many of the changes we enjoy today are accompanied by unfavorable side effects. These include chronic illnesses of many types which affect adults who feel "sick and tired" and children with ADHD and autism. Here are three of the reasons.

- *Our homes, farms, schools and other public buildings are contaminated with pesticides and other toxic or potentially toxic chemicals.*
- Antibiotics given repeatedly to many people kill friendly germs while knocking out enemies. Yeasts and abnormal bacteria multiply, leading to a "leaky gut." Food allergens and toxins are then absorbed which adversely affect the nervous system and other parts of the body.
- People are consuming nutritionally deficient, processed and packaged foods loaded with sugar, hydrogenated or partially hydrogenated fats, coloring and other additives.

Americans Fell in Love with Chemicals

Hazardous and potentially hazardous chemicals have "been around" for decades—even centuries. After the Great Depression in the 1930s and after WWII in the 1940s, Americans fell in love with chemicals. More and more were developed each year and were hailed as signs of "progress." Here are a few of them.

* Lead and other additives were added to the gasoline of our growing number of automobiles because they helped the cars run better.
* DDT and other insecticides were sprayed in our homes and other places because people felt they helped get rid of "pesky" insects.
* Weed killers and insecticides were sprayed on the soil and crops of our farms because they seemed to help farmers raise more foods to feed our growing population and export food to other countries.

Courageous Pioneers Began to Warn Us

During the 20th "Century of Progress" Americans grew and consumed more food, drove bigger and more powerful automobiles and lived in comfortable homes (heated in the winter and air conditioned in the summer). Then a few courageous pioneers began to write about the "down side" of the deluge of chemicals being introduced into our air, soil and water.

Rachel Carson In the early 1960s in her classic book *Silent Spring,* Rachel Carson compared the threat of environmental destruction from pesticides and other environmental chemicals with the risk of nuclear war. Most Americans, including legislators, farmers and food processors, paid little attention.

Carson marshaled an impressive body of evidence and claimed that pesticides had been used carelessly, with little or no advance investigation of their effect on soil, water, wild life and man itself. She forecast that pesticides indiscriminately dispersed into the global environment would haunt us long into the future by disrupting health and ecological processes fundamental to life on earth.

Theron Randolph, M.D.   About the same time the brilliant and often persecuted Chicago internist and allergist Theron G. Randolph, M.D., reported that food and chemical sensitivities played an important role in causing health problems in many of his patients. In 1962 he published the first edition of a book entitled *Human Ecology and Susceptibility to the Chemical Environment* which described the adverse effects of chemicals on health problems affecting many people.

On the cover of the sixth (1978) printing of his book, in addition to the title, Randolph asked these questions:

+ How safe is our present chemical environment?
+ To what extent does it contribute to chronic illness?
+ How much do we know about the long-term effects of such by-products of "progress" as chemical pollutants in the air, chemical additives and contaminants in food, water and biological drugs, synthetic chemical drugs, etc.?[1]

I paid the first of a number of visits to Dr. Randolph's home, office and hospital in the 1960s and learned more about his observations. He often spent over an hour listening to what his chronically ill patients had to say. Here are the comments of one of them.

> "I seem to get along fine when I stay in my home in the country, but when I visit my daughter who lives in an apartment in the city I develop a headache and muscle aches and I feel tired. There's something about the 'smell' of her apartment that bothers me."

Randolph questioned all of his patients about their possible reaction to perfumes, paints, fabric odors, gas cooking stoves, tobacco smoke and other chemical odors. *He noted that the symptoms in over half of his patients were aggravated by chemical exposures.* Although most physicians expressed skepticism over Randolph's observations, the importance of chemical sensitivities began to be recognized by increasing numbers of health professionals.

William Rea, M.D. After graduating from medical school and preparing for a career as a cardiac surgeon, an event happened that changed Bill Rea's personal and professional life. *His home was sprayed with insecticides which made him and other members of his family sick.*

Although he gradually improved, Rea noted that he had developed a sensitivity to many environmental chemicals—chemicals that did not bother other people. I recall clearly the first time I met Rea at a medical conference in the 1970s. He brought along aluminum foil to put on the seat of his chair. Here's why: chemicals emanating from the plastic seats would trigger his symptoms.

Rea has published a number of scientific articles and written several books[2] which document the role that chemical exposures play in adversely affecting many parts of the immune system. For more information see www.ehcd.com. (See also Dr. Rea's illustration of the barrel on page 70.)

Sherry Rogers, M.D. In the early 1980s, this Syracuse, New York, physician began writing and publishing scientific articles and books about allergies and food and chemical sensitivities. Included in her many publications are a 1992 book, *Tired or Toxic?* and a 1998 book, *Depression: Cured at Last!* Here are a few brief excerpts from this book.*

> "If you think you have trouble believing that everyday chemicals found in the average home and office can make people depressed you can imagine how I felt. . . One of the

_____

*You can obtain information about Dr. Rogers' books from Prestige Publishing, P.O. Box 3068, Syracuse, NY 13220. 800-846-6687 or www.prestigepublishing.com. See also references to Rogers in my discussion of environmental molds on pages 257–260).

big problems with chemical sensitivity is that it usually does not happen dramatically or quickly, but rather insidiously: it **sneaks** up on someone. . . Furthermore, most chemical sensitivity sneaks up on a person over a period of weeks, months or years, as the detoxification system is slowly damaged.

"Occasionally there will be a dramatic sudden onset of depression, for example, when new carpeting is installed or a building is renovated or freshly painted. . . One of the worst chemicals to cause chemical sensitivity and depression is the family of pesticides. . .

"Most schools or other public buildings are pesticided in the evening, on the weekends or after hours and no one sees it. So if you come in and start feeling lousy, cranky or depressed through the day, it's unlikely that you're going to investigate the pesticide history of the building."[3]

Nicholas A. Ashford, Ph.D., J.D., and Claudia S. Miller, M.D., M.S. During the past decade, these "mainstream" professionals have discussed the role that chemical pollutants play in making people sick. Here's an excerpt from the first edition of their 1991 book *Chemical Exposures, Low Levels and High Stakes.*

"An unanticipated and unwelcome opportunity for the EPA to study the effects of air pollution first hand arose when 27,000 square yards of new carpeting were installed in the agency's headquarters in Washington, D.C. in 1987 and 1988. . . An estimated 124 of 2000 employees exposed to volatile off-gassing from the carpet became ill, exhibiting symptoms ranging from eye, nose, and throat irritation and breathing problems to nausea, headache, dizziness, difficulty in thinking, fatigue, and increased susceptibility to many exposures formerly tolerated. At least two employees quit their jobs as a result of illness. Seventeen were unable to work in their assigned spaces. Some now work at home or at other locations. Eight report new sensitivities to common substances including perfumes, auto exhaust and tobacco smoke."[4]

In a review of this book in the *Journal of the American Medical Association,* James E. Cohn, M.D., MPH, University of California (SF), commented,

> "Clinicians and policymakers would do well to read and heed the advice of this book for many of us are faced with the problems of how to best evaluate patients affected by this disorder, currently without adequate guidance about the best means of diagnosis, treatment and most important, prevention. Ashford and Miller do not give us any easy answers but do point the way out of the current quagmire of opinion and empiricism, which has hindered progress toward solving this challenge."[5]

During the 1990s interest in chronic illness caused by chemicals increased dramatically. Much of this interest was stimulated because of chronic illnesses which developed in military personnel who served in the Persian Gulf. But in spite of increasing scientific documentation of the reality of the physical causes of the illnesses of these service men and women, most physicians, including those in civilian life and the government, have said in effect, "These complaints are caused by psychological stress."

In a comprehensive discussion of multiple chemical sensitivity (MCS) in the 1998 second edition of their book *Chemical Exposures, Low Levels and High Stakes,* the authors commented,

> *"Fatigue is consistently one of the most prominent complaints of MCS patients who frequently acquire a diagnosis of chronic fatigue syndrome during their medical odyssey. . .* (emphasis added) Buchwald and Garraty (1994) explored similarities and differences among 30 patients diagnosed with chronic fatigue syndrome, 30 with fibromyalgia and 30 with MCS. Patients with either chronic fatigue syndrome or fibromyalgia frequently reported symptoms consisting of MCS.
>
> "All three groups were remarkably similar in demographic characteristics and in the presence of specific symptoms; some

60–90% were female, mean ages ranged from 41–44 years, and the mean years of education was 14.7–14.9. Not surprisingly, 87–97% of the MCS patients reported sensitivities to each of the four exposure types: air pollution/exhaust, cigarette smoke, gas/paint/ solvent fumes and/or perfumes. *Likewise, 53–67% of patients with chronic fatigue syndrome and 47–67% of patients with fibromyalgia also reported adverse effects when exposed to these substances.* (emphasis added)

"*. . . Despite the different diagnostic labels, existing data, though limited, suggest that these illnesses may be similar, if not identical, conditions . . . In fact, the diagnosis assigned to patients with one of these illnesses may depend more on their chief complaint and the type of physician making the diagnosis than the actual illness process.*"[6] (emphasis added)

John Wargo, Ph.D. In his 1996 book *Our Children's Toxic Legacy, How Science and Law Fail to Protect Us from Pesticides,* Dr. Wargo (Yale University), in discussing pesticides in foods, said,

"With every meal, we're intimately affected by the quality of the food and water we consume. The complex nature of chemicals we eat and drink may include both nutrients essential for life and other chemicals that my jeopardize our health. . .

"Some U.S. companies manufacture pesticides that the U.S. Environmental Protection Agency (EPA) has prohibited from domestic use . . . These banned pesticides, however, may reappear as residues in imported foods, a phenomenon termed 'the circle of poison' by U.S. environmental and consumer interest groups. . . Today, nearly 325 active pesticide ingredients are permitted for use on 675 different basic forms of food, and residues of these compounds are allowed by law to persist at the dinner table."

"Nearly one-third of these 'food-use' pesticides are suspected of playing some role in causing cancer in laboratory mice, another one-third may disrupt the human nervous system, and still others are suspected of interfering with the endocrine system."[7]

Concern about pesticides was also expressed by neurologist David Perlmutter of Naples, Florida, in a letter to the editor published in the April 20, 1994, issue of the *Journal of the American Medical Association*.

> "The U.S. government, hoping to stimulate the American economy, stands poised to improve the General Agreement of Tariffs in Trade (GATT).—The GATT rules would allow substantial levels of pesticide residues on U.S. imported produce. Levels of DDT, 5000% higher than current U.S. tenets would be permitted on imported peaches and bananas with similar deregulations affecting grapes, strawberries, broccoli and carrots."

Small Amounts of Chemicals May Limit or Obstruct Hormonal Activity with Potentially Serious Long-term Effects.

Although I learned from C. Orian Truss, M.D., how and why candida overgrowth could cause decreased libido, menstrual disturbances and other kinds of endocrine dysfunction, I knew little about the adverse effects of chemicals on hormones. Then in the late 1980s I met Mary Lou Ballweg, Head of the Endometriosis Association, who made me aware that PCBs and other toxins were playing a part in causing endometriosis and other endocrine and immune problems. A short time later, Pennsylvania gynecologist George Miller told me that Dr. Theo Colborn was carrying out research work on the disrupting effect of chemicals on hormones (in wildlife and in humans).

Theo Colborn, Dianne Dumanoski and John Peterson Myers
Our Stolen Future is the title of a 1996 book by Colborn, a senior scientist with the World Wildlife Fund, Dumanoski, a journalist with a special interest in global environmental issues and Myers, who works with a private foundation to support efforts to pro-

tect the global environment. Acclaim for this book came from many directions. Here are representative comments.

"A chilling account of a fascinating scientific discovery. All who are concerned with preserving the earth and the health of its children and grandchildren will find this book both important and rewarding."—Robert Redford

"It could become the biggest scientific and public relations bombshell to hit the chemical industry since Rachel Carson's 1962 classic, *Silent Spring*. . . The first book to weave decades of research on hormone disruptors into a single deserving picture.—*USA Today*

In the Foreword to this book Al Gore quoted the pioneer observations of Rachel Carson, who said:

"We're subjecting whole populations to exposure to chemicals which animal experiments have proved to be extremely poisonous and in many cases cumulative in their effects. These exposures now begin at or before birth and—unless we change our methods—will continue through the lifetime of those now living. No one knows what the results will be because we have no previous experience to guide us."

In commenting on the implications and importance of this book, Gore said,

"Although scientists are just beginning to explore the implications of this research, initial animal and human studies link these chemicals to myriad effects, including low sperm counts; infertility; genital deformities; hormonally triggered human cancers, such as those of the breast and prostate gland; neurological disorders in children, such as hyperactivity and deficits in attention; and developmental and reproductive problems in wildlife. . .

"We certainly waited too long to ask the right questions about PCB, DDT and other chemicals now banned that presented serious human health risks. . . *Our Stolen Future* is a critically important book that forces us to ask new questions about the synthetic chemicals that we have spread across this earth. For the sake of our children and grandchildren we must urgently seek the answers. All of us have the right to know and an obligation to learn."

Sheldon Krimsky   *Hormonal Chaos* by Sheldon Krimsky, a professor in the Department of Urban and Environmental Policy at Tufts University, discussed the hazards of environmental chemicals. Here are excerpts from comments on the cover of this book.

"The chemicals that have ushered in the modern industrial age are literally everywhere—in pesticides applied in ever increasing quantities to food crops, in plastic microwavable containers, in dental amalgams and in the resins that coat the inside of tin cans. For decades, such substances have generally been regarded as safe at low exposures. *But new evidence suggests that relatively low levels of industrial chemicals may mimic or obstruct hormonal activity—with potentially devastating long term effects that range from cancer and reproductive abnormalities to cognitive dysfunctions like attention deficit disorder.* (emphasis added)

"Given both the seriousness and the uncertainty of the findings, how should the science of chemical toxic allergy be revised to account for these endocrine effects? And how should the scientific debate affect public policy?

"In *Hormonal Chaos,* Sheldon Krimsky traces the emergence of an unorthodox hypothesis that casts new suspicions on a broad range of modern industrial chemicals. At the heart of his story is the environmental endocrine hypothesis, the assertion that chemicals called 'endocrine disruptors' are interfering with the normal functioning of hormones in animals and humans. The theory is both attractive and troubling—attractive because it offers a unified explanation for a wide array of ills affecting modern societies; troubling because of its staggering implication for the effects of modern industrial practices."[8]

My Comments: People who are tired develop health problems from many causes. On page xi of this book you'll find a picture of the overloaded camel and the observations cited by authorities in this chapter show clearly that the chemical "bundle of straw" is one of the heaviest.

REFERENCES

1. Randolph, T.G., *Human Ecology and Susceptibility to the Chemical Environment,* Charles C. Thomas, Springfield, IL, 6th printing, 1978.

2. Rea, W.J., *Chemical Sensitivity,* Vol. I–IV, CRC Press, Boca Raton, FL, 1992–1998.

3. Rogers, S., *Depression: Cured at Last!,* Prestige Publishing, Syracuse, NY, 1998.

4. Ashford, N.A. and Miller, C.S., *Chemical Exposures, Low Levels and High Stakes*, Van Nostrand Reinhold, New York, 1991, p. 70.

5. Cohn, J.E., Book review, *Journal of the American Medical Association*, October 12, 1991.

6. Ashford, N.A. and Miller, C.S., *Chemical Exposures, Low Levels and High Stakes*, Van Nostrand Reinhold, New York, 1998, pp. 228–229.

7. Wargo, J., *Our Children's Toxic Legacy, How Science and Law Fail to Protect Us From Pesticides,* Yale University Press, 1996/1998, pp. 4–5, 78–84.

8. Krimsky, S., *Hormonal Chaos—The Scientific and Social Origins of the Environmental Endocrine Hypothesis,* The Johns Hopkins University Press, Baltimore, 2000.

Yeasts and How They Make You Sick

What Are Yeasts?

Yeasts are single-cell organisms that belong to the vegetable kingdom and, like their mold cousins, they live all around you. One family of yeasts, *Candida albicans,* normally lives in your body and, more especially, in your digestive tract. This yeast possesses a number of unique traits, including certain animal-like characteristics. And it must consume other substances such as sugar and fats in order to survive.

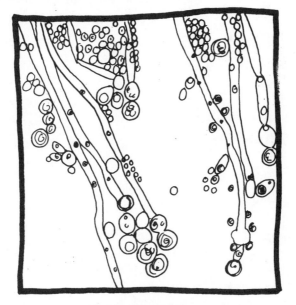

Mold Hyphae and Spores
(microscopic view)

In addition, candida has been referred to as a "Dr. Jekyll and Mr. Hyde" sort of critter. Here's why. It can switch from a single-cell yeast form into a branching fungal form. This fungal form can burrow beneath the surfaces of mucous membranes.

Yeasts Normally Live in Your Body

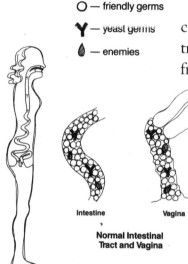

O — friendly germs
Y — yeast germs
⬤ — enemies

Intestine   Vagina

**Normal Intestinal
Tract and Vagina**

Yeasts normally live on the mucous membranes of the digestive tract and vagina. So do billions of friendly germs. Unfriendly bacteria, viruses, allergens and other enemies also find their way into these and other membrane-lined passageways and cavities. But when your immune system is strong, they aren't able to break through into your deeper tissues or bloodstream and make you sick.

When Yeasts Multiply They Produce Toxins

When you take antibiotics, especially if you take them repeatedly, many of the friendly germs in your body (especially those in your digestive tract) are "wiped out." Since yeasts aren't harmed by these antibiotics,

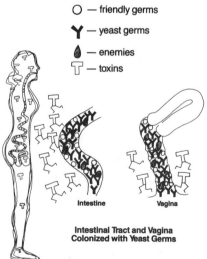

O — friendly germs
Y — yeast germs
⬤ — enemies
T — toxins

Intestine   Vagina

**Intestinal Tract and Vagina
Colonized with Yeast Germs**

they spread out and raise large families (the medical term is "colonization").

When yeasts multiply, they produce toxins. Yeast overgrowth in the gut may also play a part in causing food allergies and nutritional deficiencies.

Yeast Toxins Make You "Sick All Over"

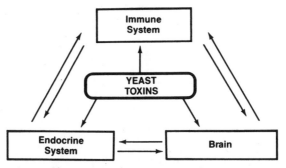

Yeast toxins affect your immune system, your nervous system, and your endocrine system. Moreover, these systems are all connected. So yeast toxins play a role in causing allergies, vaginal, bladder, prostate and other infections, as well as fatigue, headache, memory loss, depression, insomnia and other nervous symptoms. When your endocrine system is adversely affected you may develop menstrual irregularities, PMS, sexual dysfunction, infertility, sugar craving, anxiety, constipation, dry skin, low body temperature and fatigue.

About Your Immune System and How It Protects You

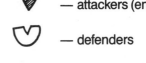

— attackers (enemies)

— defenders

— mucous membrane

Your immune system is composed of many different defenders, including white blood cells, antibodies and immunoglobulins. Some sit just under the surface of your mucous membranes*—ready to pounce on invaders.

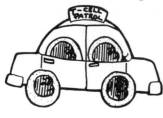

Others—including the lymphocytes (a special type of white blood cell)—circulate and patrol the deeper tissues and organs of the body a hundred or more times a day attacking and wiping out enemies that may have sneaked in.

Yeast Toxins Weaken Your Immune System

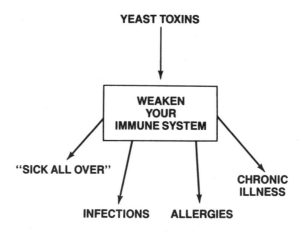

When your immune system is weak, you're apt to feel "sick all over" and develop yeast and/or fungous infections of the skin, nails or vagina.

You may also become more susceptible to viral, bacterial and other infections, and develop mold, chemical, food and other allergies, intolerances and sensitivities.

You may also develop other health disorders, including CFS, hives, psoriasis, arthritis, Crohn's disease or multiple sclerosis.

---

*Such a membrane forms the "skin" of the interior cavities of your body (mouth, nose, digestive tract, respiratory tract, vagina, etc.).

Other Factors Also Weaken Your Immune System

A viral infection may weaken your immune system. Nutritional deficiencies (caused by inadequate intake and/or poor absorption of essential nutrients) may also weaken your immune system.

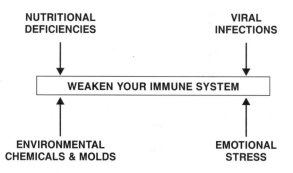

So does living or working in an environment loaded with chemical pollutants of many types.

A heavy load of environmental molds also adversely affects your immune system. So does emotional stress or deprivation.*

Every Part of Your Body Is Connected to Every Other Part

Although we sometimes seem to forget it, every part of your body is connected to every other part. So when yeast toxins and allergens affect one part of the body, they're also causing changes in other parts.

---

*As described by Ronald T. Glasser in his book *The Body Is the Hero,* 1976; Norman Cousins in his books *Anatomy of an Illness* and *The Healing Heart;* and Bernie Siegel in his books, *Love, Medicine and Miracles* and *Peace, Love and Healing.*

The "Yeast Connection"— Controversy and Support

If you review medical history, you'll find countless examples of new ideas that helped sick people get well, and that were stumbled on "accidentally." Some of these discoveries were made by scientists working in their laboratories and others by practicing physicians. Still others were made by nonphysicians. *But regardless of who makes a discovery, or what the discovery is, if a full scientific explanation of the mechanism isn't forthcoming, it tends to be rejected by the establishment.*

This seems to be the situation with the "yeast connection." Here's a summary of the story.*

C. Orian Truss, M.D., a board-certified internist, first observed in the early 1960s that the common yeast *Candida albicans* could be related to fatigue, depression and many other systemic and nervous symptoms. During the next 15 years, Truss found that many of his patients with complex medical problems responded to a low-carbohydrate diet and nystatin, an oral antifungal medication.

---

*Material in this chapter was adapted from a 24-page booklet, A Special Message for the Health Professional published by the International Health Foundation in August 2000. Copies of this booklet can be obtained from IHF, Box 3494, Jackson, TN 38303. A donation of $10 is requested.

Word of the Truss experiences spread to a handful of physicians at a medical conference in Toronto in 1977. Subsequently, he published his observations in 1978, 1980, 1981 and 1984 in the *Journal of Orthomolecular Psychiatry.** Because this journal was not peer reviewed, Truss' observations were not available in medical libraries and most physicians remained unaware of them.

One of Truss' patients, Diane Thomas, wrote an article in the early 1980s entitled "New Hope for Allergy Patients," which was published in *Atlanta Magazine* and subsequently in *Inn America* (a publication of the Holiday Inn Corp.). In 1983 Truss published his observations in a book entitled *The Missing Diagnosis.*† Included in the book are three of his papers published in the *Journal of Orthomolecular Psychiatry.* Here are their titles: "Tissue Injury Induced by *Candida albicans*," "Restoration of Immunologic Competence to *Candida albicans*," and "The Role of *Candida albicans* in Human Illness." The Truss observations were also discussed in a health food magazine and on a popular interview program, the Freeman Report (CNN).

During the 1980s millions of people all over the world learned about the relationship of *Candida albicans* to fatigue, depression, PMS and other symptoms through reports in the press and media and through popular books, including *The Yeast Connection* and *The Yeast Syndrome.*

Skepticism and Controversy

Although a few brief reports were published in the peer-reviewed medical literature, the relationship of *Candida albicans*

---

*Journal of Orthomolecular Psychiatry, 7375 Kingsway, Burnaby, B.C., V3N 3B5. Present journal name, *Journal of Orthomolecular Medicine.*

†To obtain information about this book write to *The Missing Diagnosis,* Box 26508, Birmingham, AL 35226.

to fatigue and other disorders was rejected by the medical establishment. For example, in a report on what they termed "the candidiasis hypersensitivity syndrome," the Practice Standards Committee of the American Academy of Allergy and Immunology (AAAI), stated,

- "The basic elements of the syndrome would apply to almost all sick patients at some time
- "The complaints are essentially universal:
  a. The broad treatment program will produce remission in most illnesses regardless of cause.
  b. There's no published proof that *Candida albicans* is responsible for the syndrome.
  c. Elements of the proposed treatment program are potentially dangerous."[1]

An identical statement was sent to members of the American College of Allergy, Asthma and Immunology. A "negative" commentary was also published in the *Journal of the American Medical Association (JAMA)*.

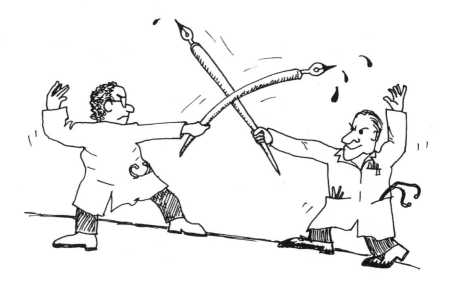

During the past 15 years the controversy has continued. On one side, there are a few thousand professionals who have found that a special diet and antifungal therapy helps many of their patients. On the other side are a much larger number of physicians who continue to say in effect, "The yeast connection is a fad disorder."

The Dismukes Report and the Bennett Editorial

In the December 20, 1990, issue of the *New England Journal of Medicine,* William E. Dismukes and associates of the University of Alabama published findings of a "randomized, double-blind trial of nystatin therapy for the candidiasis hypersensitivity syndrome." They evaluated a group of women with vaginitis who complained of fatigue, depression, PMS and other symptoms. *In treating them, they only used oral and vaginal nystatin. They made no changes in diet and in their opinion, their results were "negative."*

In an accompanying editorial, "Searching for the Yeast Connection," John E. Bennett, M.D., of the National Institute of Allergy and Infectious Diseases, Bethesda, Maryland, said,

> "Few illnesses have sparked as much hostility between the medical community and a segment of the lay public as the chronic candidiasis syndrome. Those who argue for the existence of this complex of symptoms . . . have leveled a serious charge against the medical community, claiming that it is not fulfilling one of its most important obligations to its patients. The charges simply put: You physicians are not listening to your patients. . . . Physicians pay more attention to the patient's normal laboratory test-results than to what the patients say. . . .
>
> "Even more damaging is the profession's apparent refusal to study chronic candidiasis. How can science reject an idea that has not been tested when science is purportedly open to new ideas?"

In his continuing comments, Bennett said,

" . . . Those who argue for the existence of the chronic candidiasis syndrome will complain that diet was not controlled and that it is an important aspect of treatment. . . In addition, candida allergy shots, injunctions to avoid moldy environments, and other therapeutic approaches are often included in treatment regimens. In fact, *none of the proponents of the syndrome have recommended the use of nystatin alone and they are not likely to consider the Dismukes study an adequate test of their hypothesis*. (emphasis added)

" . . . The study by Dismukes is only a beginning. Additional scientifically sound studies will be needed to determine whether this syndrome does or does not exist and if it does, what the optimal treatment is for patients."[2]

Responses in the
New England Journal of Medicine

A number of professionals took exception to the Dismukes observations and wrote letters to the editor of the *New England Journal of Medicine* and to other publications. Some were published and some were not. Here are excerpts of several letters published in the May 30, 1991, issue of *NEJM*.

"We see, in these data, strong support for the proposal that generalized symptoms caused by toxins or other mechanisms may accompany mucosal yeast infections."

C. Orian Truss, M.D., and associates
Birmingham, AL

"I challenge the conclusion by Dismukes et al. that the candidiasis hypersensitivity syndrome 'is not a verifiable condition.' This negative conclusion is not substantiated by the results of their clinical study, which shows a strikingly positive effect of the all nystatin regimen in women with the presumed syndrome."

Marjorie Crandall, Ph.D.
Torrance, CA

"Does (their study) mean that nystatin is of no value as part of a comprehensive program for patients with fatigue, premenstrual tension, gastrointestinal symptoms and depression? In my experience, and that of hundreds of other physicians and thousands of patients, the answer is a resounding 'No.' With few exceptions, the patient with a chronic health problem requires multimodal therapy. . . . And as noted by Bennett, 'None of the proponents have recommended the use of nystatin alone.'

"Additional scientifically sound studies are desperately needed. . . I would especially urge the investigators to look at the important role and intricacies of diet. A diet low in sugar (and other simple carbohydrates) was an essential part of the treatment program first outlined by Truss."

William G. Crook, M.D.
Jackson, TN

How Should the Efficacy
of a Therapy Be Determined?

In answering this question, I'd like to quote from a statement by the Office of Technology Assessment, Congress of the United States in 1978. In a publication entitled "Assessing the Efficacy and Safety of Medical Technologies," appeared the following comments:

"It has been estimated that only 10 to 20% of all procedures currently used in medical practice have been shown to be efficacious by controlled trials. . . . Personal experience is perhaps the oldest and most common informal method of judging the efficacy of a

medical technology (emphasis added) . . . It is important to point out that many medical advancements have properly and successfully proceeded without rigorous statistical methodology of evaluation."

And in an article in the *Journal of the American Medical Association,* James S. Goodwin, M.D.,* and Jean M. Goodwin, M.D., M.P.H., of the University of New Mexico said that too often an effective treatment for disease is ignored or rejected because some physicians feel that it doesn't make sense. In their continuing discussion they said,

> "Pharmaceutical companies have . . . turned to theoretical over practical arguments for using their drugs. Therefore, we're asked to use a new arthritis drug because it stops monocytes from crawling through a filter . . . and an oral diabetes drug because it increases insulin receptors on monocytes.
> "What gets lost in such discussions are the only three issues that matter in picking a therapy. Does it help? How toxic is it? How much does it cost? In this atmosphere we are at risk for rejecting a safe, inexpensive, effective therapy in favor of an alternative treatment, perhaps less efficacious and more toxic."[3]

A similar point of view was expressed by Gene H. Stollerman, M.D., in an editorial entitled "The Gold Standard."

> "As the insights of modern medical, bioscience and technology increase our medical powers, I find renewed strength in my clinical skills. Clinical experience is the 'gold standard' on which patient care should be based."[4]

Several thousand physicians in practice and a handful of academicians have found that a sugar-free special diet and oral anti-

---

*For further observations of Dr. James Goodwin, see pages 25–26, 89–91.

fungal medications are effective in helping patients with a diverse group of health problems including chronic fatigue, psoriasis, endometriosis and asthma.

Support for "The Yeast Connection"

During the mid and late 1990s a number of reports have supported the relationship of *Candida albicans* to health problems which affect many people. Here's a summary.

Asthma

Two reports on the successful use of antifungal drugs in patients with persistent asthma were published in abstract form in the January 1994 *Journal of Allergy and Clinical Immunology.* One of these reports described the observations of Belgian researchers who carried out a double-blind, placebo-controlled study on corticosteroid-dependent asthmatic patients without evidence of fungal infection. *Four out of five of the patients who received the antifungal medication (Nizoral) improved in two weeks while four out of five of those who received the placebo did not improve.*

University of Virginia researchers studied ten patients with chronic asthma and accompanying fungal infections of the feet. Fluconazole (Diflucan) was used in treating these patients. *They found that antifungal therapy was associated with overall clinical improvement, including reduction in asthma symptoms.*

In 1999 the Virginia investigators published their observations in an article entitled "Treatment of Late-Onset Asthma with Fluconazole." Here's an excerpt from the abstract of their article.

> "An improvement in symptoms, peak flow and steroid use was maintained up to 36 months after starting fluconazole in patients who continue to receive treatment. The results show

that fluconazole can be useful in the treatment of patients with severe or moderately severe asthma who have dermaphytosis."[5]

Autism

William Shaw and colleagues at the University of Missouri (Kansas City) found fungal metabolites in individuals with autism (*Clin. Chem.*, 41/8, 10/94–11/94, 1995). Following treatment with oral antifungal agents, the abnormalities improved and the children's symptoms lessened, often dramatically. Since his initial studies, Shaw has continued his investigations and has found that probiotics and dietary changes help both adults and children with other health problems, including children with the Attention Deficit Disorder.

Endometriosis

In 1996 the Endometriosis Association,* in two cover stories in their newsletter said,

> "No other approach to endometriosis treatment has given as consistent, long-term, positive results as has treatment for Candida albicans/allergy/infection and its related problems."[6]

Further evidence of the relationship of *Candida albicans* to endometriosis was published in a January 1997 issue of *Patient Care*. Here's an excerpt of an article entitled "Current Approaches to Endometriosis."

> "If the endometriosis symptoms worsen (after) receiving a small drop of *Candida albicans* under their tongue, the patient is considered allergic to the organism and in need of treatment that includes oral tolerization, antifungal drugs and proper diet."[7]

---

*Endometriosis Association, 8585 N. 76th Place, Milwaukee, WI 53223. "Endometriosis and *Candida albicans:* even more startling connections."

Chronic Fatigue Syndrome and Fibromyalgia

In 1998 Jacob Teitelbaum, M.D., and B. Bird completed a placebo-controlled study of 70 patients with fibromyalgia/chronic fatigue syndrome using multiple therapies, including the antifungal drug Sporanox. The patients in the treated group enjoyed "significantly greater benefit" when compared to the placebo group. (P=.0001).[8]

Interstitial Cystitis

During the past decade, Phillip Mosbaugh, M.D., an Indiana urologist, has treated over 500 patients with interstitial cystitis. During 1997 and 1998 he studied 15 patients with severe IC who were given multi-modality therapy including Diflucan, 200 mg daily for four months. Other treatment measures included a rigid antifungal diet, Omega-3 fatty acids, vitamin/mineral supplements and probiotics. In a May 1998 report Dr. Mosbaugh said that six patients in the study had clearly improved, some were better in some ways and some were unimproved or worse in other ways; four patients dropped out of the study for various reasons. In commenting on his study, he said,

> "These people have a lot of things on their plate. . . Bowel problems, joint aches and pains, fatigue, headache and other symptoms. . . People with these symptoms have multiple causes and multiple therapies are necessary."[9]

Multiple Sclerosis

R. Scott Heath, M.D., a Cincinnati neurologist and Kottil Ramahan, M.D., studied ten patients with MS who were treated with Diflucan and diet. In summarizing his study, Dr. Heath stated,

> "Review of our data would indicate that Diflucan does appear to show a trend in cutting the frequency of new lesions

appearing in multiple sclerosis . . . Several of the patients in the study improved and had no new lesions on MRI. These were the patients who were most compliant on their diet."[10]

Psoriasis

In letters to the editor published in the *New England Journal of Medicine* and the *Archives of Dermatology,* E. W. Rosenberg and colleagues, University of Tennessee Health Science Center, reported an association between intestinal yeast and psoriasis.[11, 12] In 1994, they published further observations. Here's an excerpt of the summary of their report.

> "Fourteen patients were treated with oral nystatin, fluconazole or ketoconazole. Nine patients were evaluated following adequate treatment. Of these, seven were cleared or substantially improved."[13]

Depression & Bipolar Disorder

During the early 1980s I kept records of 100 consecutive adult patients with yeast-related problems. Their three main complaints: *fatigue, headache and depression.* In her book, *Healing Depression—A Holistic Guide,* Catherine Carrigan* told of her 18-year struggle to overcome depression and bipolar disorder. She said, "I took the best pills, followed the advice of countless well-meaning psychiatrists . . . Despite the money, time and effort devoted to my mental health, I never knew what it meant to be mentally balanced."

Then in 1994 she received a comprehensive treatment program for chronic fatigue syndrome which included dietary changes, antiyeast medications and other therapies. During a

---

*Carrigan now holds workshops for physicians and laypeople and is head of an organization called **Total Fitness.** To learn more, look at her web page, www.totalfitness.net, send her an e-mail to daylilly@aol.com or call 404-350-8581.

recent conversation, Carrigan told me *she has been off psychiatric medications for more than five years with no relapse.*

Her story about how she overcame years of serious depression should give hope to countless people.

REFERENCES

1. *Journal of Allergy and Clinical Immunology,* 78:271–73, 1986.

2. Bennett, J., *New England Journal of Medicine,* 1990; 323:1766–67.

3. Goodwin, J.S. and Goodwin, J.M., "The Tomato Effect—Rejection of Highly Efficacious Therapies." *JAMA,* 251:2287–90, May 11, 1984.

4. Stollerman, G., "The Gold Standard," *Hospital Practice,* Vol. 2, No. 1A, January 30, 1985, p. 9.

5. Ward, G.W., et al., "Treatment of Late-Onset Asthma with Fluconazole," *J. Allergy Clin. Immunol.,* 1999; 104:541–546.

6. Personal communication, 1999.

7. *Patient Care,* "Current Approaches to Endometriosis," January, 1997.

8. Teitelbaum, J., Bird, B., *Journal of Musculoskeletal Pain,* 1996, 3(4).

9. Personal communication.

10. Personal communication.

11. Rosenberg, E. W., et al., *New England Journal of Medicine,* 308:101, 1983.

12. Crutcher, N., et al., *Archives of Dermatology;* 120:433, 1984.

13. Skinner, R.B., "Psoriasis of the Palms and Soles Is Frequently Associated with Oropharyngeal *Candida albicans,* ACTA. Derm. Venereol (Stockh.), 1994; suppl. 186:149–150.

Prescription Antiyeast Medications

Five prescription medications are now being used by physicians in North America to eradicate or control *Candida albicans* and/or other yeasts and molds—Nystatin, Nizoral (ketoconazole), Diflucan (fluconazole), Sporanox (itraconazole) and Lamisil (terbinafine hydrochloride). A sixth antifungal medication, amphotericin B* (Fungizone, Squibb), is used commonly in Europe and is now available from several pharmacies in the U.S. (These are the same pharmacies that stock nystatin powder listed later in this chapter.)

Nystatin

If your CFS is yeast connected, you'll be hearing about the antiyeast medication nystatin†. So I think you'll be interested in knowing how it was discovered and where it got its name.

You'll be especially interested if you're a woman. Here's why. Two brilliant women scientists collaborated in discovering this remarkable antifungal substance over 50 years ago. In the late 1940s, mold researcher Elizabeth Hazen and organic chemist Rachel Brown began looking for agents in the soil which might be useful in controlling fungous disease. And while working at the Albany laboratory of the New York State Health Depart-

---

*This antifungal medication is closely related to nystatin and given orally it is extremely well tolerated and is virtually non-toxic.

†Brand names include Mycostatin (Squibb) and Nilstat (Lederle). Generic preparations of nystatin are also available.

ment, they found many antifungal substances. However, most of them were toxic, not only to yeasts, but also to laboratory animals.

Then, while vacationing with friends on a farm in Warrenton, Virginia, Elizabeth Hazen dug a soil sample and took it back to her laboratory. Cultures of this soil revealed a mold that kept other molds (including *Candida albicans*) from growing. Moreover, tests showed that this mold did not harm the animals. These scientists named their discovery after New York State, nystatin (NY-Stat-In).

In 1951, Hazen and Brown signed an agreement with E. R. Squibb and Sons to study the drug, patent it and produce it. In their agreement with Squibb, royalties were put in a special scientific and educational fund. Neither of these women asked for or received personal financial gain from their discovery.

Nystatin was marketed exclusively by Squibb until 1974 and since that time has been manufactured and marketed by other companies. During the decades after its discovery it was used mainly in suppositories to treat vaginal yeast infections. And not until the reports of C. Orian Truss in the late 1970s was it used to discourage yeast growth in the intestinal tract.

Then, during the decade of the 1980s, physicians began using oral forms of this medication along with a sugar-free special diet in treating patients with fatigue, headache, depression, PMS and other symptoms.

The dosage forms for oral use are tablets, capsules, liquid solutions and powder. Although the tablets are convenient and easy to obtain on prescription, I usually recommend the nystatin powder. Here's why.

1. Yeasts live in your digestive tract from your mouth to your anus. Accordingly, the powder helps you get rid of

yeasts in your mouth, esophagus and stomach, as well as in your intestines.

2. The powder contains no food coloring, chemicals, dye or other similar ingredients that may cause reactions in chemically sensitive patients.

3. The powder is more economical.

I like nystatin for a number of reasons. Here's one of them. It is perhaps safer than any medication a physician can prescribe for his or her patients. According to the *Physician's Desk Reference* (which gives information on over 2,500 prescription drugs), "Nystatin is virtually nontoxic and nonsensitizing, is well tolerated by all age groups, even on prolonged administration."

Here's a major reason for the safety of nystatin—very little is absorbed from the intestinal tract. Accordingly, it helps a person with yeast-connected CFS by controlling candida growth in the intestinal tract.

The usual starting dose is 500,000 to 1 million units, four times a day. (Each tablet equals 500,000 units; ⅛ teaspoon of powder equals 500,000 units.) *Your own health professional will decide on the dose.* During the late 1990s and in 2000, Dr. Truss told me that a number of his patients needed much larger doses of nystatin (4,000,000–8,000,000 units, four times a day.)

If your pharmacy does not stock powdered nystatin, you can fill your prescription from one of the pharmacies listed on page 183 of this book.

Systemic Anticandida Drugs
(Nizoral, Diflucan, Sporanox and Lamisil)

Nizoral, the first of these systemic antifungaldrugs became available on prescription in the U.S. in 1981. Diflucan* and

---

*You'll find more information about long-term Diflucan therapy on pages 177–179.

Lamisil were approved by the FDA in the early and mid 1990s. This approval was given only for limited use in fungal infections, vaginal yeast infections, nail fungal infections and for people with AIDS and other serious diseases caused by weakness of the immune system.

However, thousands of physicians in practice (including a number I've consulted during the mid and late 1990s) have found these medications safe and highly effective in helping people with many chronic disorders, including chronic fatigue, psoriasis, interstitial cystitis and headache. *The decision as to which of these drugs should be used, the dose and duration of therapy, must be decided by your own personal physician.*

Pfizer has created the Diflucan Patient Assistance Program to assist uninsured patients. Eligible patients who have no insurance coverage and meet designated income criteria can receive Diflucan free. For more information, patients should contact their health professional and have that individual apply on their behalf.* (Phone 800-869-9979.)

During the fall, winter and spring of 1999/2000 I interviewed a number of physicians who are interested and knowledgeable in treating patients with fatigue and other yeast-related disorders. Here's a summary of what I learned.

+ These drugs are the "first team" and are indicated for patients with chronic fatigue who give a history of repeated antibiotics and symptoms which indicate that their health problems are yeast-related.
+ Appropriate diagnostic studies should first be done to rule out other causes of the patient's symptoms.
+ *These antifungal medications, while highly effective, are only*

---

*Based on reports I've received from a number of clinicians whose patients have received compassionate supplies of Diflucan, the clinical diagnosis of gastrointestinal candidiasis may be used.

one part of an effective treatment program and until, and unless, the patient also makes changes in her diet, the antifungal medication will not be effective.

+ Avoidance of environmental pollutants is an essential part of any anticandida treatment program.

+ Although choice of medication used and duration of use varies, the majority of the physicians I interviewed rank Diflucan at the top of the list.

+ Duration of therapy: The medication should be continued on a daily basis for 2–4 weeks or longer, until improvement occurs. Then the dose may be reduced to every other day or less often. *The decision will be made by your own physician and will depend on your medical history and your own unique requirements.*

+ If the initial antifungal drug is not effective, a different antifungal drug may be prescribed.

+ Some physicians use a systemic drug in the initial treatment of their patients, while others prescribe nystatin initially and follow it up with a systemic drug.

+ Other physicians advocate combined therapy using nystatin and a systemic drug. Here again your own physician will decide and make appropriate recommendations.

+ *Adverse reactions: Any drug regardless of how "safe" it appears to be can cause adverse reactions either mild or serious.* Because I experienced adverse reactions to several prescription drugs which I've taken during the past 40 years, I am extremely conservative. I do not recommend a prescription medication if I feel there are safe alternatives.

Nevertheless, I feel that taking these prescription antifungal drugs if indicated based on your medical history, is much safer than allowing your health problems to go untreated. I repeat, no drug provides a "quick fix" for candida-related health problems. You must also consume an appropriate diet and take other measures to overcome your fatigue and other symptoms.

✦ Die-off reactions: Most people who take prescription (or nonprescription) antiyeast medications feel worse for several days after taking them. Symptoms include fatigue, depression, aching, irritability and abdominal pain. Yet when they continue their medication, their symptoms disappear. Such symptoms are due to "die-off" reactions. Here's what seems to be happening. When the medications kill large numbers of yeasts in your digestive tract, metabolic products are released. Until your body gets rid of them, your symptoms may continue to increase.

To lessen the possibility of such reactions, follow a strict diet for a week before taking the antiyeast medication. Such a diet features vegetables, lean meats and eggs and avoids sugar, corn syrup, honey, fruit, grains and processed foods.

More About Long-Term Diflucan Therapy

In the mid-1990s, the late R. Scott Heath, M.D., and Kottil Ramahan, M.D., carried out a study on ten patients with multiple sclerosis (MS) who were treated with a program which featured dietary changes and Diflucan. In reviewing their data, Dr. Heath stated that Diflucan appeared to show a trend in reducing the frequency of new lesions in MS patients. Four of the patients in the study improved and had no more lesions on MRI. *Those who improved were most compliant on their diets.* The dose of Diflucan used in this study was *200 mg each day for 120 days.**

Another clinical study to evaluate possible yeast influences in interstitial cystitis (IC) was carried out on 15 IC patients by Phillip G. Mosbaugh, M.D, an Indiana urologist. The study

---

*This dosage is greater than those discussed on the package insert, which only mentions FDA approved indications.

which began in May 1997 was completed in June 1998. In May 1998 Dr. Mosbaugh in a letter to me said, "Six patients in the study had clearly improved. Some of the other patients were better in some ways and unimproved or worse in other ways."

The dose of Diflucan used was the same as that used in the MS study: 200 mg each day for four months. No adverse or toxic reactions were reported.*

Here's more. Dozens of people write and call the International Health Foundation (IHF) seeking names of a health professional who will prescribe oral antifungal medications. Much to my regret, few physicians are interested in seeing patients with yeast-related problems. So I was pleased and excited to receive a letter from a Colorado woman (I'll call her Suzanne) in May 2000. Here are excerpts from her letter.

> "Thank you for your help in finding a physician in my area who is knowledgeable about yeast and its effects on the body. I found a doctor in the Denver area about a half an hour drive from my home who's on my HMO. I've been taking 200 mg of Diflucan for about six weeks with remarkable results. My most troublesome symptoms were fatigue, vaginal discharge, pain with intercourse, a multitude of digestive problems, more and stronger allergies and lack of libido. . .
>
> "I feel I've had great success so far staying on a strict diet and taking Diflucan. My allergies have decreased significantly, my asthma has improved tremendously, I'm now jogging. I no longer need ten hours sleep. I've had no digestive symptoms for quite some time. Thank you from the bottom of my heart for your help. If I can be of any further assistance please let me know."

In early June 2000, I received another letter from Suzanne. Here are excerpts.

---

*You'll find a further discussion of the MS and IC studies in the International Health Foundation booklet, *A Special Message to the Health Professional* (see page 160 for ordering information) and in the 2000 printing of *The Yeast Connection Handbook*.

"I'm quite excited to report that I keep getting better! My doctor has taken me off of Diflucan after only nine weeks. She's overjoyed by my progress. I'm now taking nystatin four times a day and continuing on the diet. Though I'm allowed to cheat a bit. . . Regarding my previous letter, by all means use it in your next book. Whatever you feel will help get the message out to others feeling the same way I did. You have my permission to use all of my correspondence as you see fit. . .

"I started having asthma symptoms about ten years ago when I was in my late 20s. Even then, my allergies were getting out of control. . . I also started wheezing from seemingly unnoticeable smells. This scared me. I went to a doctor and was told it wasn't a big deal, just allergenic asthma. . . I started reading about asthma. Most of the mainstream books say, 'Once you get it you'll have it for life. . .' The wheezing frightened me so I stopped exercising. I had recurrent bouts of bronchitis off and on for four years as I got weaker and weaker.

"I picked up a copy of your book, *The Yeast Connection Handbook,* at a local health food store. It was like I was reading my own life story. I wrote to the International Health Foundation for help and found the name of a wonderful doctor from the list you sent me. There really isn't much to tell after that. JUST A SHORT, SWEET, SIMPLE RECOVERY AND MY LIFE BACK!

"I'm jogging—Colorado Springs is 10,000 plus feet above sea level. I hiked up to 10,500 feet last weekend and jogged back down. . . I can go down to my basement and look at old moldy comic books. I have tons of energy with only 7–8 hours sleep instead of the previously required ten plus. *The list goes on and on. It's as if the last ten years of my life never existed.* I realize you've heard this many times before. Yet, I cannot help but say it again—thank you Dr. Crook! Treating the yeast has completely changed my life."

As you might guess, Suzanne's letters made me happy. But they also made me feel sad. Here's why. Few physicians, like the board-certified Colorado gynecologist, are knowledgeable and experienced in using antifungal medications in helping their patients with fatigue, headache, depression and other chronic disorders.

I hope this situation will change—and change rapidly—in the next several years. Here's why. University of Virginia researchers published their findings in a major allergy journal in 1999 describing their success in using Diflucan in treating patients with chronic asthma and accompanying skin fungal infections.[1] Based on this report I hope that other researchers will carry out studies using antifungal medications and dietary changes in asthma patients who *do not* have skin fungal infections.

In a series of articles published in the June 1998 SUPPLE-MENT to the *Journal of the American Academy of Dermatology,* researchers from a number of university centers reported their success in treating toenail fungal infections with fluconazole (Diflucan), given once a week in varying doses for a period of six months. (The doses used were: 100, 300 or 450 mg.)

The following results were reported by Lynn A. Drake, M.D., and colleagues at the Massachusetts General Hospital, Boston.

> "Fluconazole was significantly superior to placebo in eradicating clinical and mycologic symptoms of onychomycosis both at the end of active treatment and at 6 months after treatment."[2] ($p = .0001$ for all efficacy measures.)

Fungi and Sinusitis

In 1999, Jens U. Ponikau and colleagues at the Department of Otorhinolaryngology, Mayo Clinic, Rochester, MN, published a study which showed that "fungal cultures of nasal secretions were positive in 202 (96%) of 210 consecutive CRS (chronic rhinosinusitis) patients. . . Allergic fungal sinusitis was diagnosed in 94 (93%) of 101 consecutive surgical cases with CRS based on histopathologic findings and culture results."[3]

Although in these two latter reports the investigators described no systemic symptoms, I hope that their observations and the University of Virginia study will lead to a further studies of the role *Candida albicans* and other fungi play in causing health problems in various parts of the body.

REFERENCES

1. Ward, G.W. et al., "Treatment of Late Onset Asthma with Fluconazole," *J. Allergy Clinical Immunology.*, 1999; 104:541–6.

2. Drake, L. A., et al., SUPPLEMENT to *Journal of the American Academy of Dermatology,* Vol. 38, No. 6, Part 2, June 1998, pp. 87–94.

3. Ponikau, J.U., et al., "The Diagnosis and Incidence of Allergic Fungal Sinusitis," Mayo Clinic Proc., 1999; 74:877–884.

Nonprescription Antiyeast Agents

Before writing this chapter, I consulted licensed health professionals, pharmacists and other knowledgeable consultants. I obtained a tremendous amount of helpful information. Experiences and recommendations were diverse and interesting. Almost without exception, all emphasized the importance of a low-sugar diet and probiotics, and pointed out that none of these agents provide a "quick fix." Miklos Boczko, M.D., a Scarsdale, New York, physician was among my consultants. And he said,

> "Answering your questions about these agents isn't easy because of the tremendous individual differences both in tolerance and benefit."

In Chapter 43 of *The Yeast Connection* (published in 1986), I discussed caprylic acid, garlic and *Lactobacillus acidophilus*. These three nonprescription agents were the *only* ones that I knew about which help control yeast overgrowth in the digestive tract. Then in the late 1980s and early 1990s, I received information from many sources which showed that other nonprescription agents were effective, including citrus seed extract, Tanalbit and taheebo tea (Pau d'Arco). I included a reference to these and other products in my books published in the 1990s, including *Chronic Fatigue Syndrome and the Yeast Connection, The Yeast Connection and the Woman* and *The Yeast Connection Handbook*.

Several other books published in the 1990s, including the *Encyclopedia of Natural Medicine* (Michael Murray, N.D., and Joe

Pizzorno, N.D.) and the 1,068-page book _Alternative Medi-cine—The Definitive Guide_ (Burton Goldberg Group) described other nonprescription antiyeast medications. So did _The Scientific Validation of Herbal Medicine_ (Daniel B. Mowery, Ph.D.). Included in these books was a discussion of goldenseal, Oregon grape, barberry, rosemary, tea tree oil and licorice.

Then in the mid and late 1990s, I received information about other nonprescription agents from patients, health professionals and pharmacists. I included a brief discussion of two of these products, oregano and undecylenic acid, in the Postscript of the 1999 and 2000 editions of _The Yeast Connection Handbook_ (pages 251–252).

I also included a paragraph on olive leaf extract and Kolorex, a herbal product derived from a New Zealand plant. To gain more information about these products, I sent questionnaires to a number of health professionals who treat their patients with yeast problems and to several pharmacies who distribute nonprescription yeast remedies.

Here's a discussion of several of these products.

Olive Leaf Extract
(OLE)

Although I've had no experience in using OLE,* I've received favorable reports from people who have called and/or written

---

*OLE is produced and marketed by many companies. It is available from An Ounce of Prevention, Englewood, CO (Fax: 303-843-9188; e-mail: annron@advcontools.com) and a number of pharmacies including the Apothecary, Bethesda, MD (800-869-9159), College Pharmacy, Colorado Springs, CO (800-888-9358), Freeda Pharmacy, New York, NY (800-777-3737), Hopewell Pharmacy, Hopewell, NJ (800-792-6670), NEEDS, Syracuse, NY (800-634-1380), Wellness Health & Pharmaceuticals (800-227-2627),Willner Chemist, New York, NY (800-633-1106) and Women's International Pharmacy, Madison, WI (800-279-8011). If you would like more information about OLE, get a copy of Dr. Walker's concise but comprehensive book, _Olive Leaf Extract_.

me. I was also impressed by the information in Dr. Martin Walker's 1997 book, *Olive Leaf Extract*. Then in the spring of 2000 I received additional information from Stan Meyerson, a pharmacist and president of NEEDS, Syracuse, New York. Here's a brief summary of what I have learned about OLE.

It is made from the leaves of olive trees and contains plant pharmaceuticals, including *oleo oleuropin,* a potent antimicrobial which inhibits the growth of any microorganisms, including viruses, bacteria, protozoa, fungi and yeast. Here are two testimonials.

> "I was troubled with multiple symptoms, some of which were back and neck pain, flu, flu-like symptoms, swollen glands, sinus and digestive problems. I was subsequently diagnosed with fibromyalgia (chronic fatigue syndrome) and the physicians recommended Prozac-type antidepressants and anti-inflammatory drugs, but I refused them.
>
> "On a treatment program which included olive leaf extract, three tablets four times a day, plus vitamin and mineral supplements, my overall health has greatly improved and so has my energy and disposition. . . I would highly recommend East Park™ Olive Leaf Extract to anyone with fibromyalgia (chronic fatigue syndrome)."

Another testimonial came from Janelle Goodman who had taken the olive leaf supplement for one month. Here are excerpts from her letter addressed "To Whom It May Concern."

> "For the last few years I have not been feeling like myself. I've had little energy and enthusiasm for anything. . . My head was always achy and I couldn't figure out why. I started taking olive leaf extract and noticed an immediate elevation of my spirits. . . After a few days I began to notice more energy and a stronger sense of well being. . . It was amazing to see the fatigue disappear and my general health improvement. I couldn't believe that I felt so well."

My Comments: During the spring of 2000, two physicians I talked with said in effect,

> "Although we continue to prescribe Diflucan and other antifungal drugs for many of our patients, we've found that a sugar-free special diet and olive leaf extract help, especially in follow-up therapy."

Kolorex

According to Irv Rosenberg, PD, a nutritional pharmacist at the Apothecary in Bethesda, Maryland, this product is as effective as nystatin. Rosenberg sent me a copy of an article by Arnold Fox, M.D., entitled "Kolorex: The New Cure for Candida." Here are excerpts.

> "From New Zealand comes a successful easy-to-use, non-toxic and natural product that effectively treats candida infections. In the cold, damp parts of New Zealand's vast forest there's a shrub called the *Pseudowintera colorata*, which has been used medicinally for centuries by the indigenous people, the Maoris. The Maoris taught early European settlers how to use the plant.
>
> "More modern study of the *Pseudowintera colorata* reveals that it contains a very powerful antifungal substance called *polygodial*. When mixed with the traditional South American medicinal plant which contains *anethole*, Kolorex has proved to be a powerful agent in the fight against candida.
>
> "Kolorex damages the cellular walls of *Candida albicans* (as well as other yeasts). With their walls ruptured, candida's cellular material leaks out and the organism dies. Kolorex kills candida more rapidly and effectively than most medicines.

In discussing Kolorex, Rosenberg, who has been counseling yeast patients for the past 17 years, said,

"It comes in a capsule form. The usual dosage is one capsule a day for five days in order to lessen the amount of die-off reaction. Then, I recommend it twice day for 8–12 weeks. It is also available in a cream for topical/vaginal use.

"Before starting this medication, I put my patients on a special diet which eliminates sugar, yeast products, yeasty foods and fruits for 4–6 weeks."*

Undecylenic Acid

Fatty acids have been known and used for centuries as antimicrobial agents, originally in the manufacture of soaps. The last 50 years, however, they have found uses both *in vitro* as yeast and mold inhibitors in foodstuffs and as topical, intestinal systemic antifungals. One of these fatty acid products, caprylic acid, has been used successfully by many health professionals and their patients during the past two decades.

In March 2000, Ann Fisk, R.N., who owns a small company, An Ounce of Prevention in Englewood, Colorado, told me about another fatty acid product, undecylenic acid, an 11-carbon mono-unsaturated fatty acid occurring naturally in the body in perspiration. According to information I received from Thorne Research, Inc.,† *undecylenic acid has been shown to be approximately six times more effective as an antifungal than caprylic acid* (emphasis added). This company produces and markets SF722 which contains undecylenic acid in a base of olive oil.

Ann Fisk also told me about another product containing undecylenic acid: Undecyn®—the calcium salt of undecylenic acid. According to information I received from Thorne Research, fatty acid salts are more sensitive to pH than fatty acids, and calcium undecylenate needs to be delivered to the intestinal tract

---

*You can find more information about Kolorex on the internet at www.forestherbs.co.nz-capsules.htm.

†Fax 303-843-9188; e-mail: annron@advcontools.com.

at an acid pH. Undecyn® contains betaine hydrochloride, which is gradually liberated throughout the intestinal tract, grapefruit seed extract and bentonite clay.

Research articles sent to me by Thorne Research included an August 1945 article published in the medical literature from a section on dermatology at the University of Chicago which reported favorably on the use of undecylenic acid in the treatment of skin fungal infections.* A second article from the University of Chicago published in 1955 discussed the effect of short chain fatty acids on yeast metabolism.†

In July 2000 I also interviewed Terry Chappell, M.D., Bluffton, Ohio, and asked him about his experience in treating his patients with the undecylenic acid product SF722. Here are excerpts.

> **WGC:** When you see a new patient who comes in saying, "I've read Dr. Crook's book *The Yeast Connection Handbook,* I've had lots of tests, been to many physicians and I flunked the quiz in front of his book. I feel certain my health problems are yeast related." What do you do first after you've carefully reviewed the patient's history and carried out tests you feel are appropriate?

> **TC:** I will start with the diet and antifungal therapy with the first visit. If they are really sick, sometimes I'll put them on the diet before I start the antifungal therapy, but that's not really very often. Usually I start them on SF722, acidophilus and the diet.

In our continuing discussion Dr. Chappell told me that he used other diagnostic methods and therapies, including muscle testing and homeopathic dilutions of *Candida albicans* that he

_____

*P.O. Box 25, Dover, ID 83825, 208-263-1337, fax: 208-265-2488. E-mail: ninfo@ thorne.com.
†*Arch Dermatology Syphilol,* 1945; 52:166–171.

found effective. His sources include Bio Energetics, Inc., 800-334-4043; BioActive Nutritional, Inc., 800-288-9525; and Viotron International, 800-437-1298.

I also talked to the naturopathic physician Dr. Bruce Blinzler of Coeur d'Alene, Idaho. He told me that SF722, along with acidophilus and diet, was effective in helping almost 90% of his yeast patients. He said,

> "I put my yeast patients on the program for one month. Then I have them come back in. I would say 80–90% of the time, as long as they stick to the diet very strictly and take the medication, their problems usually clear up . . . unless they've had a yeast problem for a long time or a very severe case."

David Schlesinger, Licensed Acupuncturist/Medical Herbalist, of Santa Barbara, California, who specializes in treating candida-related ailments, also provided me with information about SF722. In our long discussion, Schlesinger told me that SF722 causes a yeast-cleaning effect on the gut and he often uses it "as a support remedy." He said,

> "Other remedies which are capable of passing into the systemic circulation including Biocidin, a product made by a California company, Bio Botanical Research, may be needed in patients with more difficult problems. This product contains many antifungal/antiparasitic ingredients, including gentania, golden seal and sanguinaria. Your readers can find more information on my web page www.modernherbalist.com."

Garlic

Garlic has been widely used for medicinal purposes for centuries. For example, Virgil and Hippocrates mention it as a remedy for pneumonia and snake bite. In looking through the *Index Medicus,* I found numerous articles from American and foreign literature describing the inhibitory action of garlic on candida organisms.

In studies carried out several years ago, Dr. Benjamin Lau of Loma Linda University, Loma Linda, California, reported on the effectiveness of Kyolic aged garlic extract against _Candida albicans_ infections in mice. According to Dr. Lau, this study suggested that the garlic extract strengthens the immune system by helping the body's white blood cells gobble up enemy germs.

As you probably know, many different garlic products, including odor-free garlic, are available from health food stores. Like the various automobile makers, each company describes the features of their garlic products. Which preparations are best? I don't know. Yet, I've been impressed by reports that document the quality of Kyolic aged garlic extract. Over 200 peer-reviewed studies have confirmed its efficacy.

Tanalbit

Several health professionals I've consulted ranked Tanalbit high on the list of nonprescription substances they use in treating their patients. When taken orally this product is said to effectively destroy harmful bacteria and fungi in the digestive system without attacking friendly organisms. In addition to natural tannins, this product contains zinc. It comes in bottles of 60 capsules and the suggested use is 1–2 capsules a day.

Tannates are said to be effective because they act through agglutinating/astringent effects. They bind irreversibly to lipoproteins and lectins on the surface of the fungal membranes. As a consequence, the fungal cell loses its ability to adhere to the host's epithelial membrane and the ability to colonize. The tannate covered surface blocks fungal metabolism, and agglutinates them. Rapid atrophy of the fungal membranes follows resulting in the death of the fungal cell.

Tanalbit can be obtained from many pharmacies and health food stores, including The Apothecary (800-869-9151), N.E.E.D.S (800-634-1380), and Wellness Health & Pharmaceuticals (800-227-2627). You can also order it from the Internet, www.healthestores.com or from www.immunesupport.com. It can also be ordered from Scientific Consulting Services, 466 Whitney St., San Leandro, CA 94577 (650-632-2370).

Oregano

I first heard about this perennial pungent herb of the mint family from Ann Fisk, R.N., a member of the Advisory Board of the International Health Foundation. A short time later, Jeffrey S. Bland, Ph.D., discussed oregano in the September 1996 issue of *Preventive Medicine Update*. I obtained further information in an article by Robert A. Ronzio, Ph.D., and colleagues.

Based on the scientific studies presented in this article, these researchers concluded that oregano is an effective antiyeast agent and more potent than caprylic acid.

I've also received favorable reports from several health professionals who are using oregano in treating patients with yeast-related disorders. To obtain additional information I consulted Jonathan Wright, M.D., Kent, Washington. He told me that he had found oregano to be a safe and excellent antiyeast agent. Moreover, he said that in his experience it was as effective as nystatin. His usual dose: one 50 mg tablet four times daily.

Information about a special emulsified form of oregano (A.D.P.) can be obtained from Biotics Research, P.O. Box 36888, Houston, TX 77236. (Fax: 281-240-2303; 800-231-5777.)

Citrus Seed Extract

Like nystatin and caprylic acid, this antifungal agent discourages the growth of *Candida albicans* in the intestinal tract. I first heard about the efficacy of citrus seed extract in controlling candida from Drs. Leo Galland and Charles Resseger. Both said that citrus seed extract is as effective as nystatin and caprylic acid and other nonabsorbed antifungal agents in treating patients with the Candida Related Complex. It is also effective against giardiasis and some of the other intestinal parasites.

A number of health professionals I've talked to recommend Tricycline, a product that combines grapefruit seed extract and the herbs artemesia and berberine.

ParaCan

In February 2000 I received information about this natural product which incorporates a blend of herbs that have been used for decades to eliminate microbes and worms. Its main active ingredients include black walnut hulls, wormwood, pumpkin seed, Pau d'Arco, echinacea, barberry, gentian, garlic, olive leaf, cloves, chamomile and thyme.

I've also received reports from other sources that several of the herbs contained in this product help control the overgrowth of *Candida albicans* and other yeasts in the digestive tract. According to the web page, www.genhealth.com, "ParaCan . . . is an effective and . . . safe way to achieve optimal internal health. However on some occasions where parasitic activity is high, some individuals may experience nausea, weakness or fatigue during the cleansing process."

Although this product is not now available in health food stores in the U.S., it can be ordered from Genesis Health Marketing in Australia. Fax: 612-9663-5310; e-mail: sales@gen health.com.

Comments by Others

James H. Brodsky, M.D., a long time friend and author of the Foreword to my 1986 book *The Yeast Connection* and my

1995/1998 book *The Yeast Connection and the Woman,* made the following comments in a July 2000 letter to me.

> "I still recommend Tanalbit for patients who are not doing well with nystatin and/or Diflucan. I do not usually recommend nonprescription antifungals during the first month or two of prescription therapy. For those patients who are not doing as well as expected by the end of the second month, I recommend the addition of Tanalbit, 2–3 tablets, three times daily with meals. Other nonprescription antifungals that I use include caprylic acid, garlic, grapefruit seed extract and olive leaf extract, 500 mg, 1 to 3 times daily.
>
> "I've found olive leaf to be more helpful than other nonprescription antifungals. It is also useful for viral illnesses and helps boost immune function in patients with chronic fatigue syndrome."

In June 2000 I had a long phone visit with Jodi Smith, Brownsburg, Indiana, a diet and nutritional consultant and a member of the Advisory Board of the International Health Foundation. Here are brief excerpts from what she told me about how she helps people with yeast problems who consult her.

Smith emphasized the importance of changing the diet and rebuilding the immune system. She said people with the yeast problem need to understand the extreme importance of the total picture rather than just taking antifungal medications. In our continuing discussion she said,

> "The first question you asked me is what nonprescription antifungal medication I found most effective. Again, I take the theory that the yeast is able to mutate and may become resistant to antifungals. So I stay away from products that contain a large variety of antifungals. *I try to use one thing at a time.* I start my clients out on garlic to get them acclimated to the diet and understand what die-off is like. Then I've used very successfully in some people oregano oil, grapefruit seed extract,

olive leaf extract, and of course the prescription antifungals as well.

"But to repeat, I recommend one agent at a time and if the person is working with the physician and their problems are severe, I feel that Diflucan for two weeks would be appropriate. Then they can follow up with a nonprescription antifungal for a month, and perhaps nystatin for a couple of months. What I find is that people tend to get on an antifungal and they seem to have results if they stay on it for long periods of time. Based on my experience, they may not be getting the benefit they need. That's the reason I recommend a variety of antifungals used sequentially."

Others who provided me with information included Carol Englender, M.D., Newton, Massachusetts, who uses a variety of antifungal agents. Her favorites included citrus seed extract, caprylic acid, oregano, Tanalbit, goldenseal, olive leaf extract and aged garlic extract (Kyolic).

Dr. Jill Stansbury, Battleground, Washington, in response to my questions said, *"Diet! Avoid sugar, flour, bread, pasta, junk and give lots of fiber and fresh vegetables."* She also listed a number of the nonprescription agents.

Pharmacist Larry Stevens of Wellness Health and Pharmaceuticals said that some of their customers have found Tanalbit, garlic and Biocidin helpful in controlling their yeast problems.

Concluding Comments

1. If you're fortunate, and a kind, caring, knowledgeable, interested professional is working with you, be guided by his/her recommendations.
2. If you've experienced adverse reactions to any antifungal agent, check with your health professionals. Such symptoms may be temporary (a "die-off" reaction).

3. *No antifungal agent will help you if you do not change your diet and take other measures I've described in this book.*

4. If an antifungal agent doesn't seem to be helping after three weeks, a different one may be more effective.

5. If your yeast problems are not responding to nonprescription agents, you may get more help from a prescription medication. My own first choice is Diflucan. (See also pages 177.

6. *If you are following carefully the recommendations in this book, and you aren't improving, check with your health professional to make sure that other causes of your symptoms have not been overlooked.* (See also a discussion of tests on pages 289–290.)

REFERENCE

1. Stiles, J.C., Sparks, W. and Ronzio, R.A., "The Inhibition of *Candida albicans* by Oregano," *J. Applied Nutrition*, 1995, 47:96–101.

Food Allergies

Unusual reactions to substances in a person's diet or environment have been recognized for thousands of years. Yet, it wasn't until 1906 that the term "allergy" was coined by the Austrian pediatrician Clemens von Pirquet. He put together two Greek words—*allos* meaning "other" and *ergon* meaning "action." To von Pirquet *allergy* meant altered reactivity.

Today, most doctors feel that allergy means "hypersensitivity to a specific substance, which in a similar quantity doesn't bother other people." Incidentally, that's the definition you'll find in Webster's New World Dictionary. However, if you move from one city to another, you may run into different ideas about allergy—how it is defined, how it is diagnosed and how it should be treated.

Most of my colleagues in the major allergy organizations have felt that the term "allergy" should be limited to those conditions in which an immunological mechanism can be demonstrated using skin tests or more sophisticated laboratory tests. But today there are many allergists with impeccable personal and academic credentials who are emphasizing the importance of food allergies/sensitivities which can be demonstrated by using elimination/challenge diets.

Included among these physicians are William T. Kniker, University of Texas, Joseph A. Bellanti, Georgetown University, and Sami Bahna, University of South Florida. Each of these physicians discussed food allergies and sensitivities at the November 1999 conference *ADHD: Causes and Possible Solutions.*

Types of Allergies

When you develop an allergy to something you breathe, such as grass, pollen, animal danders or house dust mites, the cause of your symptoms can be suspected from your history and identified through the use of the simple allergy scratch test. In carrying out such a test, a physician scratches or pricks your skin and applies a small amount of an allergy extract.

If you're allergic to the test substance in the abstract, as for example Bermuda grass, ragweed or cat dander, within a few minutes an itching bump or welt that looks like a mosquito bite will pop up on your skin.

Skin testing will usually produce similar welts if you're allergic to foods such as eggs, peanuts or strawberries. However, if you're obviously sensitive to these foods, skin tests aren't needed to identify them. Moreover, skin testing of foods that have caused severe reactions can be dangerous.

There are other types of food allergies and sensitivities you need to know about. Such allergies have been called "hidden," "masked," "variable," or "delayed-onset" food allergies. *Allergies or sensitivities of this type are caused by foods you eat every day.* You'll probably be surprised to learn that you're apt to be sensitive to some of your favorite foods, especially wheat, corn, milk, yeast, chocolate, citrus and coffee.

Moreover, you may be "addicted" to foods that make you tired or develop headaches, muscle aches or nasal congestion. Like the cigarette or narcotic addict, you may feel temporarily better after you've eaten some of the foods to which you're allergic.

Controversy over Allergy

Many subjects are controversial, including religion, politics, education, abortion and many others. Food allergy is another such controversial subject. Here are comments from the Preface of a comprehensive book, *Food Allergy and Intolerance,* which was favorably reviewed in the *Journal of the American Medical Association*.

"As all who deal in the field will know, food allergy is an exciting, challenging, exasperating and sometimes controversial subject. Its study should be a clinical science with diagnosis based on a combination of clinical observations and scientific investigations. . .

"There has been a strong tendency for the conventional physician to say that if the mechanism is not understood then food allergy does not exist. . . This is of course unacceptable . . . To make a diagnosis (of food allergy) certainly requires clinical skill, but does not necessarily need a complete understanding of a mechanism underlying the disease process or an exact understanding of the etiology. . .

"*. . . the cornerstone of diagnosis of food intolerance is the removal of that food from the patient's diet, with concomitant improvement (or not) of the patient's symptoms and their reappearance on adding that food back.*"[1] (emphasis added)

Why People May Develop Adverse Food Reactions

In the August 24, 1991, issue of *The Lancet* (Vol. 338, pages 495–96), Dr. J. O. Hunter, FRCP, Addenbrooke's Hospital, Hills Road, Cambridge, CB2 2QQ, UK, presented a hypothesis to explain the mechanisms that take place in many people who experience adverse food reactions. Here are excerpts from his commentary.

"Specific food intolerance has been implicated in many conditions. In controlled trials, exclusion diets are effective in migraine, irritable bowel syndrome, Crohn's disease, eczema, hyperactivity and rheumatoid arthritis."

Yet, Hunter pointed out, because no evidence of the classical Type I allergic reaction can be found in most patients with food sensitivities, many investigators conclude that those who say, "I'm bothered by food allergies," are merely neurotic. In his discussion, he suggests that patients with food intolerance have an abnormal gut flora even though pathogens are not present.

In his concluding paragraph, he stated,

"Much further work, especially studies of gastrointestinal enzyme concentrations and of the colonic flora, is required to substantiate this hypothesis. However, if food allergy is not an immunologic disease, but a disorder of bacterial fermentation in the colon, it might be more appropriately named an 'entero-metabolic disorder.' This is of more than mere terminological importance: modern microbiology has opened the way to the manipulation of bacterial flora to allow the correction of food intolerances and thus the control of disease."[2]

An American clinician and researcher, W. Allan Walker, M.D., Professor of Pediatrics, Harvard Medical School, has carried out extensive research on the digestive tract. Here are brief excerpts of some of his comments.

"There's increasing experimental and clinical evidence to suggest that large antigenically active molecules can penetrate the intestinal surface not in sufficient quantities to be of nutritional importance, but in quantities that may be of immuno-logical importance.

"This observation could mean that the intestinal tract represents a potential site for the absorption of bacterial break-down products such as endotoxins and enterotoxins, proteolytic and hydrolytic enzymes or other ingested food antigens that normally exist in the intestinal lumen."[3]

My Comments: What goes on in the gut is important. No doubt about it! According to my mentor and friend Dr. Sidney

Baker, your intestinal tract has a surface area as large as a tennis court. During the last decade the observations of Hunter and Walker have been confirmed by many other clinicians, professionals and researchers, including Jeffrey Bland, Ph.D.

Here's the bottom-line message. *If you're tired and are sensitive/allergic to foods, antifungal medications and a sugar-free special diet will help you—sometimes dramatically.*

REFERENCES

1. Brostoff, J. and Challacombe, S., *Food Allergy and Intolerance,* London, Balliére Tindal, and Philadelphia, W. B. Saunders, 1987.

2. Hunter, J.O., *The Lancet,* Vol. 338, August 24, 1991, pp. 495–496.

3. Walker, W.A., in Brostoff and Challacombe, *Food Allergy and Intolerance,* London, Balliére Tindal, and Philadelphia, W. B. Saunders, 1987, pp. 209–222.

Elimination Diets

Almost without exception every person with a yeast-related problem is bothered by food allergies and sensitivities. *To identify the foods that contribute to your symptoms you must carefully plan and properly execute a trial elimination/challenge diet.* Here's an edited transcript of a tape-recorded visit with one of my patients.

Q: I've been tired ever since I had "mono" three years ago. I've also been bothered by headaches, muscle aches, poor memory, abdominal pain and a year-round stuffy nose. I'm wondering if my symptoms are food-related and I'd like to try an elimination diet. Please explain.

A: On such a diet you eliminate many or all of your favorite foods. To make things easier for you I have prepared two diets. The first of these—a less restrictive diet—I call Diet A. Then there's a much tougher Diet B, which I call the "Caveman Diet."

Q: I believe I'd like to try Diet A first. What foods can I eat on this diet?

A: You can eat any meats but bacon, sausage, hot dogs or luncheon meats; any vegetables but corn; any fruits but citrus. You can also eat rice, rice crackers, plain oatmeal and the grain alternatives amaranth and quinoa (obtainable from health food stores).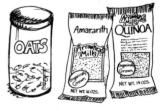

Q: Anything else?

A: Yes. Nuts in shell or unprocessed nuts of any kind.

Q: That doesn't sound too difficult, although it'll take careful planning to carry out the diet. What can I drink?
A: Water. I especially recommend bottled or filtered water.

Q: What foods do I need to eliminate?
A: Many of your favorite foods. Here's why: _The more of a food you eat, the greater your chances of developing an allergy to that food._ Here's a list of foods you must avoid on Diet A.

dairy products	orange
cane and beet sugar	egg
wheat	chocolate
corn and corn syrup*	yeast
honey	apple†
maple syrup	

This diet also eliminates food coloring, additives and flavorings which are found in many packaged and processed foods.

Q: How do I get started on a diet? What do I do first?
A: Discuss the diet with family members, prepare menus and purchase food you'll eat on the diet.

Q: Tell me more about the diet.
A: The diet is divided into two parts:
  1. Eliminate a number of your usual foods for 5–7 days and see if your symptoms improve.

---

*High fructose corn sweetener is the major ingredient of colas and other beverages.
†If you eat an apple or drink apple juice more often than once week.

2. IF and when your symptoms show *convincing* improvement, eat the eliminated foods *one food per day* and see if your symptoms return.

Q: How will I know the diet is really making a difference?
A: Buy an 8 x 10 notebook and keep a careful record of your symptoms.

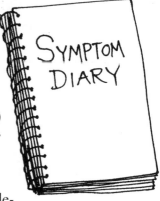

a. for three days (or more) *before beginning the diet*
b. *while you're following the elimination part of the diet* (five to ten days—occasionally longer)
c. *while you're returning foods to your diet*—one food per day

You'll need, of course, to keep a detailed record of the foods you eat.

Q: How will I feel on the diet?
A: During the first two to four days of the diet, you're apt to feel irritable and hungry and you may not feel satisfied even though you fill up on the permitted foods. You may feel restless and fidgety or tired and droopy. You may also develop a headache or leg cramps.

You may be "mad" at the world because you aren't getting the foods you crave, especially sweets. You may act like a two-pack-a-day smoker who quit smoking "cold turkey." Here's why. People who suffer from hidden food allergies are often "addicted" to the foods causing their problems.

Here's some good news. If the foods you've avoided are causing your symptoms, you'll usually feel better by the fourth, fifth or sixth day of the diet. Almost always, you'll improve by the tenth day. Occasionally, though, it'll take two or three weeks before your symptoms go away completely.

Q: If I improve on the diet, what do I do then? When and how will I return the foods to my diet?

A: *After you're certain that you feel better and your improvement has lasted for at least two days, return the foods to your diet— one at a time.* If you're allergic to one or more of the eliminated foods you'll usually develop symptoms when you eat the foods again.

Q: What symptoms should I look for?

A: Usually, but not always, your main symptoms will reappear. In your case you're apt to feel more tired and depressed; and you'll probably develop a headache or your nose will feel stopped up. However, sometimes you'll notice other symptoms, including some that had not bothered you previously—such as itching, coughing or urinary frequency.

Q: How soon will these symptoms appear after I eat a food that I'm sensitive to?

A: The symptoms will usually reappear within a few minutes to a few hours. However, sometimes you may not notice a symptom until the next day.

Q: When I return a food to my diet does it make any difference what form the food is in?

A: Yes! Yes! Yes! Add the food in pure form. For example, pure whole wheat rather than bread, whole milk rather than ice cream, since ice cream contains sugar, corn syrup and other ingredients.

Here are suggestions for returning foods to your diet.

Egg: Eat a soft- or hard-boiled egg (or eggs scrambled in pure safflower or sunflower oil).

Citrus: Peel an orange and eat it. You can also drink fresh-squeezed orange juice (do not use frozen or canned orange juice as they are loaded with yeasts.)

Milk: Use whole milk.

Wheat: Get whole wheat from the health food store, add water and cook it in your microwave.

Food coloring: Buy a set of McCormick's or French's dyes and colors. Put a half teaspoon of several colors in a glass. Add a teaspoon of mixture to a glass of water and sip on it. If you show a reaction, you'll need to test the various food dyes separately. Red seems to be the most common offender.

Chocolate: Use Baker's cooking chocolate or Hershey's cocoa powder. You can sweeten it with a little liquid saccharin (Sweeta or Fasweet). Eat the powder with a spoon or add it to water and make a chocolate-flavored drink.

Corn: Use fresh corn on the cob, pure corn syrup, grits or hominy. Eat plain popcorn. Don't use microwave popcorn because it contains other ingredients.

Sugar: Get plain cane sugar. Perhaps the easiest way to do this is to eat sugar lumps or add the sugar to a glass of water. Do the same with beet sugar.

Q: I think I understand. I wonder if you have other things you'd like to emphasize.

A: Here are a few of them.

+ Carefully review all your instructions. Plan ahead. Don't start your diet the week before Christmas, Thanksgiving or some other holiday.
+ If you don't feel significantly better on your diet in 5 to

7 days,* eat your favorite foods—even pig out. If your symptoms worsen (including your headache, fatigue, irritability or stuffiness), chances are they're food related and you'll have to do further detective work to identify the troublemakers.

✦ Here's a suggested order for returning foods to your diet.

1. Egg	4. Citrus	7. Milk
2. Yeast	5. Corn	8. Sugar
3. Wheat	6. Chocolate	9. Food coloring

✦ Eat a small portion of the eliminated food for breakfast. If you show no reaction, eat more of the food for lunch and for supper and between meals too.

✦ *Keep the rest of your diet the same while you're carrying out the challenges.* Here's an example. Suppose you eat egg on the first day of your diet and show no reaction. Does this mean you can continue to eat egg? No. Eat egg only on the day of the challenge and don't eat it again until you've tested all the foods and the diet has been completed. The same principle holds when you test other dietary ingredients.

✦ If you show no symptoms after adding a food the first day, add another food the second day, eating all you want—unless you show a reaction.

✦ If you think you develop symptoms when you add a food but aren't certain, eat more of the food until your symptoms are obvious. *But don't make yourself sick.* If you show

---

*If you fail to improve substantially on an elimination diet, you may be reacting to offending substances in your living and work environment (exhaust fumes, paint fumes, insecticide sprays, carpet odors, etc.). Accordingly, before beginning your diet, clean up your home environment. You'll find detailed instructions on pages 68–73.

an obvious reaction after eating a food, such as stuffiness, cough, irritability, nervousness, drowsiness, headache, stomach ache, flushing or wheezing, don't eat more of that food. Wait until the reaction subsides (usually 24 to 48 hours) before you add another food.*

✦ If a food really bothers you, shorten the reaction by taking a teaspoon of "soda mixture" (two parts baking soda and one part potassium bicarbonate; your pharmacist can fix up this mixture for you). Or dissolve two tablets of Alka Seltzer Gold† in a glass of water and drink it. A saline cathartic such as Epsom salts will also shorten your reaction by eliminating the offending foods from your digestive tract.

Q: Thank you for those explanations. They make sense. Although I hope I won't have to do it, tell me a little bit about that "Cave Man Diet."

A: Okay. Here's why we call it the "Cave Man Diet." *On this diet you avoid every food you eat more than once a week! Carrying it out requires careful planning and preparation, shopping and execution.*

Here's what you CAN eat and drink on this diet.

✦ Meats: fish and seafood, lamb, shrimp, cod, salmon, other fish, lobster, scallops, wild game
✦ Vegetables: any but corn, white potato, tomato and legumes.
✦ Oils: sunflower, safflower, walnut, olive or canola.
✦ Grain alternatives: amaranth and quinoa.

---

*If you suffer from severe asthma or swelling, the food challenges should be supervised by your physician and carried out in his office or clinic.
†Alka Seltzer Gold contains no aspirin.

+ Nuts: filberts, walnuts, almonds, pecans.
+ Beverages: mineral water or spring water.

Q: Whew! I can see that diet will be tough. Will I be able to get enough to eat?

A: Yes. Although early on you'll probably suffer food cravings. But you can eat as much as you want of the allowed foods. Bake and broil your meats and fish and steam your vegetables. You can also obtain many of the calories you need from unprocessed nuts and the grain alternatives.

Continue the "Cave Man Diet" for 5–7 days, just as I recommend for Diet A. As soon as you show significant lessening of your symptoms lasting two days, start eating the foods again. This time we do it differently. Add the foods _one at a time_ at breakfast, lunch, supper and bedtime, four times a day. Eat the food in large quantities, for example, four eggs for breakfast, two baked potatoes for lunch, perhaps a whole chicken for supper and four bananas at bedtime.

If a food causes a reaction, take a laxative to get it out of your digestive tract. You can also take Alka Seltzer Gold. Delay additional food challenges until your symptoms subside.

Q: I hope I won't have to do that diet but I'd like to ask you some more questions. Can I follow the diet and still work? Can I go out or accept an invitation to eat with friends?

A: Yes. If you "brown bag" it. And if you're invited out to dinner, tell your host or hostess that you're on a "crazy diet." You can eat before you go or decline the invitation and ask for a rain check.

Q: Suppose I complete the diet and note obvious reactions to a couple of foods. Yet, there are other foods I'm not sure about. What do I do then?

A: *Keep the foods that cause a reaction out of your diet for at least a month before you try them again.* You can go ahead and re-test foods you're uncertain about. Here's one way you can do this. Eat the suspected food several days in a row; for example, Friday, Saturday, Sunday, Monday and Tuesday.

Then, eliminate the food for the next five days and after this period of elimination, load up on the food on the sixth day. If you're allergic to it, you should develop symptoms. If you show no symptoms, chances are you aren't allergic to that food.

Q: Suppose I show a definite reaction to a food—a really convincing one. Does this mean I'll *always* be allergic to the food?

A: Yes. To some degree. Your symptoms will nearly always return if you consume as much of the food as you did before you began your diet. But here's a word of encouragement. *If you avoid a food you're allergic to for several months, you'll usually regain some tolerance to it, and you may not develop symptoms unless you eat it several days in a row.*

Q: What you're saying seems to make sense, but I have another question. Why does the food bother me on some occasions and not on others? For example, I've heard of people who became congested when they drank milk in the wintertime, but could drink it in the summer without showing symptoms.

A: It has to do with the allergic "load" of other allergens. Part of the problem relates to chilling. Also, wintertime furnaces stir up dust and dry up the respiratory membranes and lessen a person's resistance and make her more susceptible to wintertime infections and allergies.

Q: How about allergies to hay fever caused by grass, ragweed or cat dander? Do they have anything to do with the amount of an allergy-causing food I can eat?

A: Yes. *The more allergy troublemakers you're exposed to, the greater are your chances of having an allergy flare-up.*

Q: I'm beginning to understand more about hidden food allergies, but suppose I'm allergic to egg and avoid it for three months. Then I eat an egg for breakfast and it doesn't bother me. How will I know how much and how often I can eat egg in the future?

A: I'm glad you asked. It will give me a chance to talk about the *rotated* diet. I've found that my allergic patients who rotate their diets usually get along well and develop fewer new food allergies.

Rotating your diet means eating a food only once every four to seven days. So if you're allergic to egg, after avoiding it for several months, you can try eating it once a week and see if you tolerate it. You can do the same with other foods.

Is there anything else you'd like to ask?

Q: Nothing I can think of at the moment. My head is spinning! Do you have further instructions?

A: Read, review and study all the instructions I've given you. You may also wish to read other books about hidden food allergies and sensitivities. When you've finished, you'll find that tracking down hidden food allergies won't be as hard as you thought it would be.

You'll find more information about rotated diets in the following publications.

- Crook, W.G. and Jones, M.H., *The Yeast Connection Cookbook,* Professional Books, Inc., Jackson, TN 38305.
- Crook, W.G., *Tracking Down Hidden Food Allergy.* Professional Books. Available from Wellness Health and Pharmaceuticals, Birmingham, AL. 800-227-2627.
- Dumke, N.M., *Allergy Cooking with Ease.* P.O. Box 4123, Lancaster, PA 17604.
- Golos, N. and Golbitz, F.G., *If Today Is Tuesday, It Must Be Chicken,* 1981. Available from Human Ecology Research Foundation of the Southwest, 12110 Webbs Chapel Rd., Suite 305, East, Dallas, TX 75234.
- Jones, M.H., *The Allergy Self-Help Cookbook,* Rodale Books, Emmaus, PA 18098.
- Lewis, S.K., *Allergy and Candida Cooking—Made Easy.* Canary Publications, P.O. Box 5317, Coralville, IA 52241–0317.
- Rockwell, S., *Cooking With Candida Cookbook* (Revised). P.O. Box 13056, Seattle, WA 98103.

Psychological Factors

During the past decade I've received thousands of letters from people seeking information and help, and other letters from people who told me how they overcame their health problems. Many who wrote to me said, "Without any question, prayer played a key role in enabling me to regain my health."

In the early 1990s I heard a presentation by Dr. Larry Dossey, author of *Healing Words: The Power of Prayer in the Practice of Medicine*. In this book, Dossey told of his initial skepticism about the possible effects of prayer; yet after reviewing dozens of scientific articles which showed that prayer could have an important influence in healing, he incorporated prayer into his medical practice.

He pointed out that people can pray for themselves or they can pray for others. He cited three studies where *people who didn't know they were being prayed for showed significant improvement, as compared to people who weren't prayed for*. And he pointed out that this was a "double blind" study. The doctors and other hospital personnel didn't know which patients were being prayed for; neither did the patients.

In answering the question, "Why does prayer work?" Dossey pointed out that there are countless examples in medical history about treatments used because they were effective—whether the mechanism could be explained or not.

During the 1990s, Dossey published several other books, including *Space, Time and Medicine* and *Reinventing Medicine— Beyond Mind/Body to a New Era in Healing* (1999). My daughter Nancy gave me a copy of this book for Christmas and I found it fascinating. Here are excerpts from the flyleaf of *Reinventing Medicine*.

"Dr. Dossey provides the scientific and medical proof that the spiritual dimension works in healing. Citing the work of scientists in such well know institutions as Princeton, Harvard and Stanford, he conclusively demonstrates that spiritual tools such as intercessory prayer, dreams, coincidence and intuition, have measurable, powerful and profound effects on how we heal.

"His argument forces us to go beyond the practices of conventional medicine which he calls Era I, and mind/body medicine, which he calls Era II, leading us to a new dimension, the spiritual, 'nonlocal' dimension of Era III. What was viewed in the past as random or episodic events in healing are shown, through scientific evidence, to be related and connected to a higher force at work—Dossey calls this force the nonlocal mind."

In his 1998 book *Power Healing*, Dr. Leo Galland discussed "the four pillars of healing." These pillars include diet, exercise, the environment and getting rid of the internal toxins that play a part in making people sick. *His fourth pillar focuses on interpersonal relationships and how they play a part in enabling people to get well.*

I especially liked his discussion of the qualities of a caring doctor which he said that all competent physicians must possess. These include ability to listen, willingness to acknowledge the patient's ideas and feelings about their illness, ability to show empathy and willingness to offer encouragement, hope and assurance.

When people write or call me seeking a physician, here's one of the first questions I ask, "Is your personal health care professional kind and caring?" If they answer "yes," I say, "She is the best person to help you, even if she knows little about yeast-related disorders."*

You'll find a further discussion of Dr. Galland's approach in his publications on his web page, www.mdheal.org.

The late Dr. Norman Vincent Peale, a wonderful minister and a dynamic speaker, wrote a fascinating book, *Imaging* (published by Guideposts, Carmel, NY). Information on the flyleaf of this book said that Dr. Peale was a timid child who was "afraid to raise his hand in school or recite before company in his home."

At some point, Dr. Peale asked the Lord to change him and to see himself in a more positive light. *Once he began to see himself differently he realized that an image vividly conceived and stubbornly held has a reality of its own.*

In his book *Imaging,* Dr. Peale emphasizes that it consists of more than thinking about a goal, such as regaining your health— *he recommends visualizing it or seeing it with tremendous intensity.* In the concluding pages of his book, in discussing "Eight Ways to a Better Image," Peale said,

> "Well suppose your self-image isn't all it should be. Can you do something about it? Of course you can! A weak self-image is not a natural state of mind. You weren't born with it. . . . Check your external appearance. Do you look discouraged and defeated? Make yourself stand straight and tall. Put a smile where that frown was. . .

My Comments: A wonderful example of "imaging" is Venus Williams who won Wimbledon, the world's most prestigious tennis tournament, at the age of 20. When Venus was ten years old, she and her father went to Florida to see the world famous tennis champion Chris Evert and looked at her trophies. Venus

---

*A 24-page booklet, *A Special Message to the Health Professional,* published by the International Health Foundation in May 2000, may help persuade a skeptical physician to prescribe nystatin, Diflucan or other antifungal medication. (See page 82)

put her hands on the Wimbledon trophy and from that day forward she began to imagine herself as the champion and began to take the many steps needed to achieve her goal.

Here's a related story that everyone in the world knows about. As a young child, Tiger Woods and his father began to visualize the day when he would win all the prestigious championships and be acclaimed as the best golfer on the planet. His vision of where he wanted to be, plus hard work, enabled him to achieve his goal.

Probiotics

I n a five-and-a-half-page Foreword to Natasha Trenev's 1998 book *Probiotics: Nature's Internal Healers,* Michael McCann, M.D., told readers of the importance of this natural product. Here are excerpts.

"Probiotics will be to medicine in the twenty-first century as antibiotics and microbiology were in the twentieth. Physicians on the front line of medical practice increasingly recognize the limitations and complications of conventional approaches of medical practices, only one of which is the overuse of antibiotics. In this book, Natasha Trenev makes a compelling case that probiotics should be recognized not only for a wide variety of practical uses, but also as a legitimate specialty worthy of the best methods of scientific inquiry . . ."

"'Pro' meaning 'for' or 'in favor of,' 'biotics' or 'life' aptly describes this new/old method. It contrasts directly with 'anti' 'biotics' or 'killing life.' *It means giving live friendly bacteria to a patient to maintain or restore health.* (emphasis added.)

In his continuing discussion McCann tells about how he "agonized" with his patients who suffered from inflammatory bowel disease (ulcerative colitis or Crohn's disease) which he said often developed after a course of antibiotics. Although some patients with this often devastating problem seem to be temporarily "cured" by antibiotics, as soon as they were discontinued, the disease recurred. In answering why, McCann said,

"Let's take your front lawn as an example. If you killed off all of the grass with a powerful herbicide . . .what would you get? Not a nice mono-crop of 'beneficial' grasses, but a variety of weeds that you do not want. Now, instead of waiting for nature to takes its course . . . let's say you reseeded with large numbers of beneficial grass seeds. . . In 1963 . . . I tried to save money by reseeding a lawn with a stingy amount of seeds. I got mostly weeds, until I reseeded with a much larger number of seeds. Then I had a lovely lawn.

"Maybe this was a good experience for me because I was reminded of this long-forgotten suburban experiment in groundskeeping when Natasha Trenev called me to say, 'Of course your patients relapse when you stop giving the beneficial bacteria. You have to keep giving them!'"

In his continuing discussion, McCann reviewed some of his experiences when working with Drs. Robert A. Good, Sami A. Bahna and other colleagues in the Department of Immunology, All Children's Hospital in St. Petersburg, Florida. He also mentioned his subsequent work with microbiologist Robert Buck in Cleveland, Ohio. In his next to last paragraph of his Foreword, McCann said that the data now available about probiotics,

". . . should be the fertile ground for the eager young scientists of the twenty-first century, just like the great minds of the twentieth century tackled individual microbes—polio, streptococcus, pneumococcus, clostridium tetanus, and many others."[1]

In August 2000 Trenev, President of Natren, Inc., a company that produces and markets Healthy Trinity probiotic supplements, sent me information about these probiotics. She said that a recent study (which has not yet been published) shows that products produced by her company are as effective as an antifungal medication in preventing yeast vaginitis. She also said that in her experience, these products should remain refrigerated or kept cool in order to guarantee potency.

Effective Against a Viral Infection

According to a front page article published in the June 2000 issue of *Pediatric News,** two researchers who made presentations at the annual meeting of the American Society of Clinical Nutrition discussed the important role of probiotics in helping infants and young children with diarrhea caused by a rotavirus. One of the researchers, Dr. Jon A. Vanderhoof, director of the section of pediatric gastroenterology and nutrition at the University of Nebraska Medical Center, Omaha, cited studies which showed that the duration of rotaviral illness was reduced by two to three days.

The article pointed out that Dr. Vanderhoof used a *Lactobacillus GG* product called Culturelle, produced by Conagra, Inc. He also recommends this probiotic for children who receive antibiotics who have previously experienced antibiotic-associated diarrhea. (Dr. Vanderhoof is the vice president of Conagra.)

The second speaker at this same conference, Dr. Jose M. Saavedra, also discussed the use of probiotics in infants and children with rotaviral diarrhea. He said there had been at least four large placebo-controlled studies which showed the value of probiotics in treating infants and young children as compared to a control group who did not receive probiotics. The main criteria he used in determining the effectiveness of the probiotic was the shortening of the duration of the diarrhea.

A second article in the June 2000 issue of *Pediatric News* described the observations of another physician which were presented at the annual meeting of the American Society for Clinical Nutrition. In this presentation Dr. Erika Isolauri of the University of Turku, Finland, pointed out that probiotics helped pa-

---

Pediatric News is published monthly in International Medical News Group, Division of W. B. Saunders Company, 60 Columbia Rd., Building B, Morristown, NJ 07960. Editorial Offices, 12230 Wilkins Ave., Rockville, MD 20852.

tients with problems other than those in the digestive tract. The problems she discussed included patients with food allergies, Crohn's disease, arthritis and other chronic conditions.

In a prior article published in the *Journal of Allergy and Clinical Immunology*, Isolauri and her colleague, Heli Majamaa said,

> "The mucosae represent a first line in host defense. Human beings are initially exposed to numerous environmental antigens during infancy, particularly through food. . . Intestinal inflammation seems to be a predisposing factor in the increased sensitization of a subject. . . The intestinal microflora is an important constituent of the gut mucosal barrier."

In the article the researchers pointed out that the current approach in the management of food allergy is complete avoidance of foods proven to cause symptoms. In their study they found that the oral introduction of probiotics can help the host by improving the intestinal microbial balance. In so doing, this would be a useful treatment for food allergy by alleviating intestinal inflammation. In their discussion, they said,

> "The hitherto imperfect understanding of the role of food allergy in atopic dermatitis has fueled a constant debate on the optimal treatment of infants with atopic eczema and food allergies. However, well-controlled studies suggest that dietary antigens do contribute to exacerbation of atopic dermatitis, at least in a subset of patients. *In these patients, as also seen in this study, an elimination diet is associated with an alleviation of clinical symptoms of atopic eczema and reversal of some disturbances in immune responses to dietary antigens.*"[2] (emphasis added)

Although the probiotic studies by U.S. researchers and those in Finland were carried out on infants and young children, I feel they are relevant to adults with chronic fatigue, especially those who give a history of infectious mononucleosis or other viral infections.

Comments of Jeffrey Bland, Ph.D.

During the past 14 years I've learned many things that I write and talk about from Dr. Bland, a tireless researcher and former colleague of the late Linus Pauling. I've also been a regular subscriber to his audio tapes which are now titled *Functional Medicine Update (FMU)*.*

In the June 2000 issue of FMU he provided his subscribers with a comprehensive discussion of the microbial contents of the gastrointestinal tract. He pointed out that a number of disorders, including inflammatory bowel disease, arthritis and spinal arthropathies are related to disturbances in gut flora. He said that we can modify the flora by giving people probiotics, one of the important constituents of his 4R™ Program;† it reinoculates the gut and helps push out parasitic bacteria by reinhabiting the gut with friendly bacteria. Here's an excerpt of his discussion.

> "We recognize that this is awakening to even the food technologists. They recently had an expert panel on food safety and nutrition in which they described scientific support for probiotics and its influence on health and function."

In his continuing discussion Bland said the importance of probiotics was also discussed in a favorable manner by Mary Ellen Sanders in the *Journal of Food Technology* (Vol. 53, page 67).

He also pointed out that there are many different strains of probiotics including the MCFM strain of *Lactobacillus acidophilus* "which has been shown to be stable and a very high adhesion. As you know adhesion is very important for replication in the gut and for these organisms to stick and actually do something."

---

*For information about Functional Medicine Update call 800-228-0622 or visit Dr. Bland's website, www.healthcomm.com.

†See pages 270–271 for additional comments on Dr. Bland's 4R™ Program.

The different forms of probiotics he discussed included some produced and sold in Sweden and other European countries, Japan and the U.S. And he said,

> "Basically what I'm saying is that there are many different forms of bifidobacteria and acidophilus that can be used as a probiotic with different adherences, different replicative rates and different personalities as to how they survive within the GI tract. *Clearly they have to be stable, they have to be able to survive GI acid and bile, they have to be able to adhere in order to be functionally able to be part of the reinoculation program. I think it's fortunate that we're seeing products being made available which deliver these characteristics. If a person doesn't respond favorably to one acidophilus or bifidobacterial product, then shift them to a different species or a different product."* (emphasis added)

Probiotics That Do Not Require Refrigeration

According to information I received from one of my consultants, Charles Fox, the Wakunaga Company, *Kyo-Dophilus,* a dairy-free product produced by his company, does *not* need refrigeration. *Kyo-Dophilus* contains three different probiotics (*L. acidophilus, B. bifidum* and *B. longum*). Each capsule provides 1.5 billion live cells. It is used in over 30,000 hospitals and clinics and is packaged in dark glass bottles. It survives stomach acids and colonizes the intestinal tract.

According to Fox, one of the advantages of this product is that it is convenient for travelers who do not have a refrigerator available. He also sent me a copy of studies from an independent laboratory which showed that this product had a three-year shelf life.[3] He also said that his company produces *Probiota,* a product which is sold in drug stores and comes in a tablet form with over 1 billion live cells and contains just *L. acidophilus.*

Comments of Beatrice Trum Hunter

During the past decade I've consulted Ms. Hunter, a nutrition authority and author of a number of books, including one on probiotics. She now serves on the editorial staff of *Consumer's Research** magazine. Here are excerpts from our recent conversation.

WGC: What is your feeling about which probiotics are best and which forms people should take?
BTH: One of them is to look for the *filtration process*. That seems to be important and should be stated on the label. That's one point.

The next point: *The company marketing the product should guarantee the number of viable colonizing bacteria*. If you do not have that assurance, you really don't know what you're getting into. Usually the number of viable colonizing bacteria is in the billions. *Then the label should also show an expiration date.*

WGC: Should probiotics be taken with meals, between meals or after meals? Does it make any difference?
BTH: Some people say to take it on an empty stomach and others say to take it with milk. Now if you happen to be milk intolerant you run into a problem. Although I feel that taking it on an empty stomach is the most effective, I don't know of any study which proves which way is best.

WGC: What are some of your other thoughts about probiotics?
BTH: It should be packaged in a *dark glass bottle*. You should instruct the patient to *refrigerate the product after it's opened*. The producers of one of the products you told me about say that their product doesn't need to be refrigerated. I don't know

---

*You can obtain more information about this organization by writing to Consumer's Research, Inc., 800 Maryland Ave., N.E., Washington, DC 20002. The magazine can be obtained by writing to Consumer's Research, P.O. Box 5025, Nashville, TN 37204–9782. ($27 a year.)

what the basis of that is, but it's probably prudent in any case to refrigerate it because if you have viable colonizing bacteria you certainly want to keep them viable.

WGC: Do you have other comments?

BTH: Yes. I'd like to point out that people who purchase commercial probiotics often don't know what they're getting. It might be simpler to tell your patients to get a *good yogurt*. A good yogurt will really help if the person can tolerate dairy products. The packets of such a yogurt should show clearly an expiration date. Yogurt that's very old is not going to be as effective as when it's fresh. However, yogurt has a fairly long shelf life.

Also get unsweetened yogurt—*just plain yogurt*. This is rather tricky. If the packet says "made with," that is not sufficient. Some of the companies heat process it after the yogurt is formed. They do that so that it has an even longer shelf life. That is not desirable. The additional heat treatment actually kills the beneficial bacteria. So the person looking for yogurt should look on the label for the phrase *"contains viable cultures"* or *"contains live and active cultures."*

In her continuing discussion Hunter said that she did not recommend frozen yogurt, which often contains sugar or aspartame. She also said that the count of live bacteria should be a minimum of two billion.

Two weeks before I completed the manuscript of this book, Hunter sent me a copy of an article in the May 2000 issue of *Food Processing*, "Beverage targets 'active people'—Drink offers fast track to intestinal tract" by Kitty Broihier, R.D., Field Editor. In her article Broihier told her readers about a new product by Dannon called Actimel. She said,

> "This is not just another fruit juice beverage . . . This is a legitimate venture into mainstreaming probiotic beverages, an already crowded nutritional beverage category . . . Actimel contains a unique combination of live and active cultures, in-

cluding 10 billion active lactobacilli casei (L. casei) cultures per 3.3-fluid ounce serving, according to Dannon product literature."

She said she tried Actimel at a recent trade show and it tastes "pretty good, with a clean, slightly tart flavor like that of plain yogurt but sweeter. It contains no artificial colors, flavors or preservatives and the product is available in supermarket dairy cases and natural food stores." The suggested retail price for a 4-pack of Actimel is $2.19.

Hunter also sent me a page from the newsletter of Stonyfield Farm yogurt which said, "This brand contains six live active probiotics cultures. You can get more information about it on the web at www.stonyfield.com.

My Comments: As I've discussed elsewhere in this book, if you're troubled by recurrent or persistent fatigue the causes are multiple, and may include a persistent low-grade viral infection which you experienced many years ago (such as a case of flu or mononucleosis). Your tired feelings may also be due to the absorption of antigens (allergens) from foods you're consuming on a regular basis; wheat, dairy products and soy are common offenders. So is corn, including corn sugar; also beet and cane sugar.

Or as I've found in my patients during the past two decades, fatigue often develops because a person has taken antibiotics from time to time for respiratory, urinary, prostate, skin or other infections, leading to an imbalance in the microorganisms in the gut.

Even if you haven't taken many antibiotics prescribed by your physician, you may be getting them in meat from chickens and other animals who are usually treated with antibiotics.

So I recommend probiotics to my patients and friends as a simple, inexpensive measure for maintaining or improving their health.

Should probiotics be given any time you take an antibiotic drug, such as amoxicillin, Keflex or Ceclor? Over the years I've said, "Yes, by all means." But in carrying out research for this book, two of my consultants said, "Wait until after the antibiotic has been discontinued until you prescribe probiotics." Their rationale, the probiotic might interfere with the effectiveness of the antibiotic in eradicating a urinary, respiratory or other infection.

A greater number of consultants said, "We always tell our patients to take probiotics *along with* the antibiotic. We know of no study which shows that this isn't the best way to proceed."

My recommendation continues to be: Take probiotics *along with* the antibiotic and for an indefinite period after the antibiotic has been completed.

REFERENCES

1. Trenev, N., *Probiotics: Nature's Internal Healers,* Avery Publishing Group, Garden City Park, NY, 1998.

2. Majamaa, H. and Isolauri, E., "Probiotics: A novel approach in the management of food allergy," *J. Allergy Clin. Immunol.*, 1997; 99:179–185.

3. Certificate of Analysis: Food Products Laboratory, Inc., Portland, OR 97220, Tim McCann, President, May 5, 1999.

Parasites

I f in spite of changing your diet, taking antifungal medications and following the other recommendations in this book you continue to feel "sick and tired," other causes of your symptoms should be investigated.

In my books published in the 1990s, I cited the observations of Dr. Leo Galland who reported that eradication of the parasite *Giardia lamblia* in the intestinal tract resulted in clearing up fatigue and related "viral" symptoms (myalgia, sweats, flu-like feeling) in many of his patients.

In discussing parasites in his 1998 book *Power Healing,* Galland said,

> "Contrary to popular belief parasitic infection is not unusual in the U.S. population. It is a common occurrence, even among those who have never left the country. Unlike bacteria, parasites appear to serve no useful function. . .
>
> "Giardia contaminates streams and lakes throughout North America and has caused epidemics of diarrheal disease in several small cities by contaminating the drinking water. One epidemic, in Placerville, California, was followed by an epidemic of chronic fatigue syndrome, which swept through the town's residents at the time of the giardia epidemic."[1]

Another parasite, *Blastocystis hominis*, also appears to be a trouble maker. According to an article in *Practical Gastroenterology* by Martin J. Lee, Ph.D.,

> "Blastocystis hominis had greater prevalence than any other parasite but often goes undetected because of poor laboratory technique. At Great Smokies Diagnostic Laboratory

blastocystis is found in 15% or more clinical specimens. The weight of evidence supports treating it as a potential pathogen."[2]

In a discussion of parasites in their book *Alternative Medicine Guide to Chronic Fatigue, Fibromyalgia and Environmental Illness,* Burton Goldberg and colleagues said,

> "Parasitic infection . . . is as difficult to diagnose as chronic fatigue syndrome itself. One of the main problems related to the study of parasitic infections and their link to systemic illness is the fact that 'most parasitology laboratories fail to find the majority of intestinal parasites in stool specimens submitted to them. . .'"

And they cited a physician from a British public health laboratory who said that parasitic infection "is almost certainly under-detected by a factor of ten or more."[3]

You'll find more information about parasites in Ann Louise Gittleman's book *Guess What Came to Dinner—Parasites and Your Health.* This comprehensive, easy-to-read and understand book will tell you with many of the things you need to know about parasites. Included will be a discussion of symptoms, diagnosis, treatment, prevention and a list of laboratories which specialize in parasitic testing. Here's an excerpt from the back cover of this book.

> "Are you having difficulty shaking off an illness? Are you suffering from chronic fatigue? Do you have health problems your doctor can't identify? Parasites in your body may be the cause."[4]

REFERENCES

1. Galland, L., *Power Healing,* Random House, New York, 1998, pp. 186–191.

2. Lee, M.J., et al., Trends in Intestinal Parasitology, Part Two: Commonly reported parasites in therapeutics, *Practical Gastroenterologist,* 1992, Vol. 16, No. 10.

3. Goldberg, B., *Alternative Medicine Guide to Chronic Fatigue, Fibromyalgia and Environmental Illness,* pp. 40–42.

4. Gittleman, A.L., *Guess What Came to Dinner—Parasites and Your Health,* Avery, Garden City Park, NY, 1993.

Free Radicals and Antioxidants

About fifteen years ago I first began hearing the terms *free radicals* and *antioxidants*. And over the years I've heard these topics discussed repeatedly by Jeffrey Bland on his monthly audio tapes, *Functional Medicine Update* (FMU).* Then in 1993, I read an 87-page book by David J. Lin, B.S., entitled *Free Radicals Shouldn't Be Free*. According to Lin,

> "Uncontrolled free radical processes may be critically involved in the cause and prevention of numerous disease conditions, conditions which before seemed unrelated."[1]

Lin noted that simple nutrients called antioxidants are perhaps the best natural defenses against harmful substances. In his continuing discussion, Lin pointed out that our bodies are constantly making them and they help our immune system destroy bacteria and viruses. He said that free radicals are important to health and it is only when they are produced in excessive amounts that they damage the body.

Free radicals are produced by many things that we eat or breathe, including cigarette smoke, rancid food, high-sugar diets, car exhaust, smog, air pollutants, pesticides and herbicides. Damage caused by free radicals can affect many parts of the body and may play a role in worsening of many serious conditions includ-

---

*Information about FMU and publications by Dr. Bland can be obtained from HealthComm International, Inc, P.O. Box 1729, 5800 Soundview Dr., Gig Harbor, WA 98335. Phone: 253-851-3943; Fax: 253-851-9749.

ing heart disease, cancer, cataracts, arthritis, Parkinson's disease and many others.

How can we cope with these free radicals? We can, of course, make appropriate changes in our lifestyle. We can stop smoking and stop polluting our homes with toxic chemicals. We can eat foods rich in the antioxidant nutrients, especially fruits, vegetables, grains and nuts. These nutrients function together as a team to quench free radicals. We can also take nutritional supplements, including beta carotene, vitamin C, vitamin E, flavonoids and reduced glutathione.

According to Drs. Allan Sosin and Beth Ley Jacobs,

> "Glutathione peroxidase (composed of the amino acids glutamic acid, cysteine and glycine) is the premier antioxidant enzyme in the body. It plays an important role in cell detoxification, heavy metal detoxification, immune function, DNA and protein synthesis, transport processes and the removal of free radicals. . . Glutathione levels tend to drop as we get older about 3–4% every decade from age 20 to 70."

In their continuing discussion, the authors stated that alpha lipoic acid (ALA) increased glutathione levels.

> "In order to perform (its) antioxidant function in the body alpha lipoic acid must be present in amounts significantly higher than normal. For the average well person, then, daily supplementation at 100 to 200 mg is sufficient as a preventable dosage. Although alpha lipoic acid is found in many foods, it would be almost impossible to obtain these amounts through diet alone. . . Some studies use daily doses as high as 600–800 mg to reverse symptoms from neuropathy."[2] (See also pages 235–236)

In his magnificent book *Detoxification and Healing—the Key to Optimal Health,* Dr. Sidney Baker said,

"One of the main points of this book is that some of the most troublesome toxins are ones that look so much like friendly molecules that they escape detection until they've already done mischief or masquerading as invited participants in a key biochemical step . . . Reduced glutathione, one of the princely members of our family of detoxification chemicals, is *lost* from the body when a foreign chemical is detoxified while it is *recovered* from detoxification operations when the toxic substances are generated from our own chemistry. . .

"Jeffrey Bland, Ph.D. . . has been and continues to be the preeminent educator of physicians whose appetite for biochemistry and immunology has been whetted by their need to study their patients as individuals. Thousands of patients have benefitted directly from the knowledge that Dr. Bland has brought to their physicians with a flawless sense for applying a rigorous, detailed understanding of biochemistry to a systems approach to medicine and a superlative knack for explaining things. . . If I have awakened your interest in the subject at hand, you'll want to read Dr. Bland's new book, *The 20-day Rejuvenation Diet Program*.

"There's no one specific way for everyone to detoxify his or her body, whether by fasting, drinking lots of vegetables juices, sweating or taking vitamins. . . There are, however, a few simple steps that apply to many people.

"The first is to avoid allergenic foods . . . The second is the use of the hypoallergenic, nutrient dense food product, Ultra Clear, designed by Dr. Bland. There are several forms of Ultra Clear and you will need some guidance in choosing the correct one. The intent of the Ultra Clear products is to support the chemistry of both phases of detoxification, as well as to help heal the bowel by providing nutrients, fiber and normal flora to the gut."[3]

REFERENCES

1. Lin, D.J., *Free Radicals and Disease Prevention*, Keats Publishing, 1993.

2. Sosin, A. and Jacobs, B.L., *Alpha Lipoic Acid—Nature's Ultimate Antioxidant,* Kensington Books, 1998, pp. 55–62.

3. Baker, S.M. *Detoxification and Healing—the Key to Optimal Health,* Keats Publishing, New Canaan, CT, 1998, pp. 39–40, 160–161.

Colostrum

According to information I've received from various sources, including the Internet, bovine colostrum provides people who take it with many health benefits. Here are several of them.

- ✦ It strengthens the immune system.
- ✦ It may help people with a "leaky gut" and food allergies.
- ✦ It may help people with inflammatory bowel disease.
- ✦ It provides growth factors.

In a research study published in the May 1999 issue of *Gut,* British researchers described studies which showed that a colostrum preparation provided major beneficial effects in gut injury by NSAIDs (nonsteroidal and anti-inflammatory drugs).[1]

Jesse A. Stoff, M.D., an Arizona physician, published a 26-page booklet entitled *The Ultimate Nutrient.* In his booklet, he described his experiences in using "antigen infused dialyzable bovine colostrum/whey extract." (AIDBCWE) He also included a bibliography with 21 references dating back to the 1970s. Sources cited included the *Journal of Infectious Diseases, Clinical Immunotherapy, Science* and *The Lancet.*[2]

Conditions which Stoff said could be helped included irritable bowel syndrome, chronic fatigue syndrome, yeast problems, sinusitis, colds, flu and several other disorders. Stoff also presented a table summarizing his experiences using colostrum in 107 patients he had seen "who presented with chronic diseases which were known to include low NK (natural killer) cell function." All of his patients were treated with a complementary medical regimen of therapy which included colostrum.

Dr. Stoff's patients were suffering from a variety of medical disorders, including chronic fatigue syndrome, allergies and cancers of various types. His "Comments on Outcome" included "remission," "much improved," "cured," "normalized," "improving rapidly," "back to work" and "full recovery."

I also received a 20-page newspaper, *Vital Health News*, which was devoted entirely to a discussion of colostrum, especially "New Zealand quality colostrum." Included in this paper were testimonials from a number of health professionals, including medical doctors (M.D.s), naturopathic physicians (N.D.s) and chiropractic physicians (D.C.s). I was especially impressed by the comments of Donald R. Henderson, M.D., M.P.H., who received a Master's Degree in public health from the Harvard School of Medicine who commented,

> "When I prescribe colostrum to patients, I clearly and routinely see them make a move toward a better quality of health and overall well being. . . Most importantly, colostrum is effective because it is such a beneficial remedy for the health of the entire gastrointestinal tract. . .   In addition to successfully combating harmful organisms . . . colostrum also encourages the colonization of beneficial bacteria in the bowel . . . As far as I can tell, there's been more solid clinical research than on almost any other natural supplement or herbal remedy."

My Comments: Every day I learn something I didn't know yesterday and it lets me know that there are many other things I need to know which might help people with chronic illness. I've had no experience in using colostrum and I've received no reports about the effectiveness of colostrum from people who have written me or from patients I've treated. Yet, based on the information cited above, colostrum supplements may help you if you're troubled by chronic exhaustion.

I hasten to add, however, that NO SINGLE NUTRIENT, vitamin, mineral or other measure you take can provide you with a "magic bullet" that will make your health problems vanish.

REFERENCES

1. Playford, R.J., "Bovine colostrum is a health food supplement which prevents NSAID induced gut damage," *Gut,* Vol. 44(5), May 1999, pp. 653–658. (http://gateway.ovid.com)

2. Stoff, J.A., *The Ultimate Nutrient,* Insight Consulting Services, Tucson, AZ, 2000.

3. *Vital Health News,* 2005 8th Ave., Seattle, WA 98121. Fax: 206-340-0145. Webpage www.bovinecolostrum.com.

Other Supplements

Alpha Lipoic Acid (ALA)

ALA is the only antioxidant which is both fat and water soluble. This means that it is easily absorbed and transported across cell membranes. However, it differs from many other antioxidants which provide only extracellular help. It is found in the leaves of plants such as potatoes, spinach, broccoli, tomatoes, carrots, yams and sweet potatoes. Meat, especially liver and heart, is also a rich source of naturally occurring ALA.

In the introduction to the book *Alpha Lipoic Acid—Nature's Ultimate Antioxidant,** Allan Sosin, M.D., one of the co-authors said,

> "In this book we'll explain how Alpha Lipoic Acid (ALA), used in conjunction with other supplements in a comprehensive program, can improve a variety of medical conditions. I've recommended it to hundreds of my patients. I'm in good health and take 150 mgs of Alpha Lipoic Acid daily to stay that way. . . Alpha Lipoic Acid is used for general health and maintenance of ideal antioxidant status in the body, in combination with other antioxidants, including vitamin C, vitamin E, CoEnzyme Q_{10} and pycnogenol."

According to Drs. Sosin and Jacobs, it has been used extensively in Europe to prevent complications associated with diabe-

---

*Sosin, Allan, M.D. and Jacobs, Beth L., Ph.D., M.D., *Alpha Lipoic Acid—Nature's Ultimate Antioxidant,* Kensington Books, 1998.

tes including neuropathy, macular degeneration and cataracts. Therapeutic applications include liver diseases, coronary heart disease, allergies, sinusitis, dry skin and many other disorders.

Barley Grass

During the past decade I've talked to people at health food conventions and elsewhere who said, "Dr. Crook, barley grass is good for you." Yet, I never followed up, until recently. In early 2000, Paula Joyner (a Nashville businesswoman whose story about her recovery from severe chronic fatigue I included in *The Yeast Connection and the Woman*), said, "Green barley really helps me keep my health and life on track." (See also pages 54–55)

Then in the April 2000 issue of *Let's Live* I read an article about barley by Rita Elkins, M.H. Here are excerpts.

"Barley grass is the product of a young, newly germinated seedlings of the barley plant. It belongs to a class of edibles called green foods, nutrient packed foods that are unusually rich in chlorophyll, the green pigment that gives plants their color. . . preliminary research suggests that barley grass may help to boost energy, fight cancer, stimulate tissue repair and even prevent coronary heart disease.

"The seed of the barley plant . . . produces a soft, lush grass that is harvested when the shoots are 10 to 14 inches high. These narrow green blades contain high concentrations of several vitamins, including vitamins A, B complex (including B12 and folic acid), C and E. The grass is also rich in calcium, iron, magnesium and phosphorous. In fact, by weight, barley grass has more than 10 times the calcium found in cow's milk, five times the iron found in spinach and seven times the vitamin C found in oranges. In addition, laboratory tests have found more than 70 other trace minerals in barley grass. As an impressive source of dietary protein, barley grass sports 18 amino acids, including the nine essential ones that can't be produced by the body."[1]

In the article, Elkins also said that research conducted at the Department of Environmental Toxicology at the University of California, Davis, showed that green barley extract helped to degrade residues of various pesticides into nontoxic substances. In a discussion on how to use barley grass, Elkins said it can be eaten fresh by making juice from the leaves or it can be purchased in powder and pill form and taken on an empty stomach about 30 minutes before or after a meal. Green barley grass powder can also be blended with fruit or vegetable juices or other supplements like wheat germ to create a "nutrient-packed" drink.

Bromelain

This proteolytic enzyme is obtained from the stem of the pineapple plant. It breaks down scar tissue, decreases edema and blocks inflammatory mediators. According to Michael Murray, in his book *The Healing Power of Herbs,* the typical dose is between 250–500 mg three times a day between meals. In his discussion he said,

> "Because of its ability to impact many aspects of inflammation it is used for people with sprains, strains, arthritis and other inflammatory conditions. . . It is especially effective alone or in combination with curcumin in reducing the need for corticosteroids in rheumatoid arthritis."[2]

Murray also said that because bromelain is a smooth muscle relaxant it has been used successfully in the treatment of other conditions, including dysmenorrhea, chronic bronchitis and sinusitis.

I received additional information about bromelain from Dale Benedict, Biotech Pharmacal, who sent me a list of references dating back to the 1950s. Included was an article which described the effectiveness of bromelain in treating patients with a variety of athletic injuries, sinusitis and rheumatoid arthritis and other problems.

According to a brochure Benedict sent me, bromelain is a prostaglandin modulator and up to 40% is absorbed when administered orally. It is virtually nontoxic. However, it should be used with caution in patients with kidney or liver problems and should not be used with patients with bleeding tendencies.

According to Benedict, Bromase (a brand of bromelain) is a superior product. He said that it contains more active ingredients than other formulations.*

MSM

This exciting substance may help you! My knowledge about this safe nutritional supplement was almost zero when I began writing this book in February 2000. At that time, a woman with yeast-related problems wrote and said, "Dr. Crook, I'm taking MSM and it helps me in many ways, including especially my headaches and fatigue."

Two weeks later, another woman who called me on my IHF hotline praised MSM. Then, a friend I saw at the golf course who knew of my interest in nutritional supplements, came up to me and said, *"Look at my hands. The pain in my fingers has gone. I can hit the ball a lot farther. I take a lot of nutrients, and the MSM is really working wonders."*

Then, in April 2000, I heard Ronald M. Lawrence, M.D., Ph.D., talk about MSM on *Larry King Live.* So I picked up a copy of *The Miracle of MSM* at my local bookstore and I've just finished reading it from cover to cover. In the chapter of this book co-authored by Lawrence, Stanley W. Jacob, M.D. and

---

*You can obtain information about this product and/or order it by calling 800-345-1189.

Martin Zucker, they told the story of Joyce Scott, who was so tired "she could hardly move" and "couldn't get out of bed."

Doctors told Joyce she had chronic fatigue and then they told her she had fibromyalgia. She also suffered from mental confusion and other symptoms, including rosaceae (a chronic red coloration affecting the skin of the nose, forehead and cheeks). After taking MSM, "the energy started to kick in and the pain started gradually going away." A month and a half after starting MSM she said she was pain-free most of the time and she called MSM, "My gift from God."

You can purchase MSM at health food stores and pharmacies, or you can order it from the Internet. But before you rush out and start taking it, get a copy of the Jacob/Lawrence/Zucker book. It's authoritative and easy to read and understand.

Here's more information about MSM. It's a sulfur-containing nutritional supplement which contains two important constituents of protein, methionine and cystine. These amino acids are present in animal proteins and plant proteins, including garlic, onions, peas, beans, sunflower seeds and many others.

According to Drs. Jacob and Lawrence, here are some of MSM's most significant actions.

+ It relieves pain.
+ It reduces inflammation.
+ It passes through the membranes of the body, including the skin.
+ It increases blood flow.
+ It provides swift relief for constipation.
+ It reduces muscle spasm.
+ It reduces scar tissue.
+ It has antiparasitic properties—especially for giardia.
+ It has immune normalizing effects.

The physician authors of this book say in effect,

"MSM is a nutritional supplement with many nurturing and health enhancing properties. If you're under treatment for any condition mentioned in this book, bring your observations to your physician's attention and obtain his/her professional opinion regarding your use of this supplement."

A Testimonial: In a letter entitled "What Works for Fibromyalgia," published in the August 1999 issue of *Let's Live,* S.B., a Gibsonburg, Ohio, woman said,

"I've had fibromyalgia for years. My husband used to say, 'No matter where you're touched, it hurts. . . You've got to do something.' I was having a hard time maintaining a normal existence. House work and yard work, for example, would cause anywhere from severe discomfort to serious pain. I didn't want to become a slave to nonsteroidal anti-inflammatory drugs (NSAIDs) so I tried some natural painkillers, including magnesium and malic acid. Nothing seemed to help much. Fortunately I discovered MSM.

"Within a week the pain was finally better and I was able to do things that I enjoy, like gardening. I'm now able to exercise 30 minutes per day, which I could not do before. I take 500 mg of MSM three times a day. While MSM may not be a cure-all, it has made life much easier for me."[3]

A personal story. In the 1970s, while running all over the tennis court trying to beat a cousin half my age, I injured the cartilage in my left knee, the joint swelled up and filled with blood. After being on crutches for a few weeks, the surgeon took out fragments. He said I was lucky the damage wasn't worse than it was. After a few months I returned to the tennis court and played doubles with people my age.

Then twenty years ago, when my knee showed a little swelling (not painful), the doctor said, "You should give up tennis and stick to golf." A couple of years ago my left knee began to give me pain. The arthroscopic and x-ray studies showed that I had "bone rubbing on bone." My orthopedist tried injections of a special substance in my knee five times. It was supposed to help. It did not. On October 13, 1998, my left knee was replaced by a skilled surgeon. No complications.

After my left knee surgery I began taking glucosamine and chondroitin. I felt they would keep me from having an operation on my right knee and would also help my other joints. Although my left knee replacement was "successful," it remained stiff and hurt when I walked up steps. So I put one foot up on a step and then put the other foot up and went up the steps slowly.

Back to the MSM part of the story. After reading about MSM, I began taking two capsules twice a day in May 2000. Since that time my knee works better. I have little pain, I can walk up steps like everyone else and I've begun to ride my stationary bicycle.

If you hurt anywhere, read *The Miracle of MSM*—it may work miracles for you.

REFERENCES

1. Elkins, Rita, M.H., "Barley Grass," *Let's Live*, April 2000, pp. 49–51.

2. Murray, M., *The Healing Power of Herbs*, Prima Publishing, Rocklin, CA 95677.

3. Jacob, S., Lawrence, R. and Zucker, M., *The Miracle of MSM*, Berkley Publishing, New York, NY, 1999.

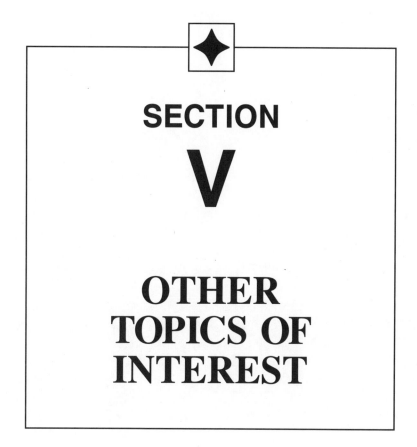

SECTION
V

OTHER TOPICS OF INTEREST

Acupuncture

Like millions of Americans, I'd occasionally develop a *severe* backache. The pain would be so bad that I could not straighten up. I'd feel like someone stuck a knife in my spine. One of these attacks came on when I stepped off a cable car in San Francisco; another came on when I was playing golf. Fortunately these episodes happen only about once every six or eight years. One afternoon, after shopping in Hong Kong, I developed one of those backaches—not the worst one I'd ever had. Although I took a hot bath and pain medication when I got back to the hotel, the back pain persisted. Now, as Paul Harvey might say, "Here's the rest of the story."

During a visit to Shanghai the week before, Betsy and I spent several hours with an American-trained Chinese allergist and his wife. During our conversations he said, "When you go to Hong Kong, look up my nephew. He's a fine young physician with traditional training who is also a skilled acupuncturist." Betsy called the young doctor, who came to our hotel to see me. While other members of our tour group looked on, he put acupuncture needles in various places on my back. I can't remember how rapidly I obtained relief, but the next day—I carried on my usual activities and my back pain did not return. (See pages 264–269)

Acupuncture for CFS and FM

According to an article by Neal Conaty, LaA.c, Dipl. Ac. (NCCAOM), published in the winter 1999–2000 issue of *Lifeline,* the quarterly newsletter of the Wisconsin Chronic Fatigue Syndrome Association, Inc.,*

---

*This article was reprinted from the August/September 1999 AACFS newsletter.

"FM and CFS are marked by global symptoms: pain in many areas of the body at once, fatigue, poor sleep and digestive disturbances to name a few. Acupuncture, with its homoeostatic effect, can be a powerful tool in combating these symptoms. . . Immediate effects of acupuncture include increased relaxation and pain relief. People often note improved sleep and digestion as well. With continuing treatment, FM and CFS flares can become less severe and less frequent . . ."With acupuncture treatment, patients are often able to work with their physicians to reduce dosages of difficult medications and sometimes eliminate the need for some. Since acupuncture is virtually without side effects, these gains are not offset by other unwanted symptoms.

"It is important the acupuncturist has the experience dealing with chronic conditions and that they are comfortable communicating with a physician and the other practitioners in the health care team."[1]

Acupuncture: *Is It for You?*

This was the title of a three-page article in the January 2000 issue of *Fibromyalgia Network* (a newsletter for people with fibromyalgia syndrome/chronic fatigue syndrome) written by Kristin Thorson; based on a speech by Miles Belgrade, M.D., a neurologist and acupuncturist from Minneapolis.*

"Unlike many other alternative medicines," says Belgrade, "acupuncture does have a scientific foundation that is consistent with the Western scientific thinking in pain medicine biology. The evolution of our understanding of endorphins—the pain fighting chemicals produced by the body—has helped acupuncture move forward in its scientific basis. . .

---

*For information about this article write to FIBROMYALGIA NETWORK, P.O. Box 31750, Tucson, AZ 85851-1750. Phone: 800-853-2929. Fax: 520-290-5550. Website, www.fmnetnews.com.

"Acupuncture was introduced into the United States when President Nixon opened China to the West and we sent over a team of ping-pong players. One of the players, James Reston, fell ill with appendicitis. He had his appendix removed under general anesthesia, but his post-op pain treatment consisted of acupuncture. Reston was so impressed with the effectiveness of acupuncture that he wrote an editorial that appeared on the front page of the *New York Times* in 1972."

In answering the question, "What is acupuncture?," Dr. Belgrade said,

"It's a form of stimulation of the body to achieve a therapeutic goal . . . The stimulation can be from needles penetrating the skin; it can be in the form of heat; or it can be in the form of laser or pressure stimulation. The key is that there is a defined set of points being stimulated."

The editor of *Fibromyalgia Network* mailed out questionnaires to 400 subscribers to FM Network in Washington State to learn how they rated acupuncture. Here are some of the responses.

+ 43.7% excellent/good; 13.5% fair; 25.1% not improved/poor; 17.7% unsure.
+ Number of visits required before noting an improvement, 3–4.
+ The average cost per visit was $50/an hour.
+ The top symptoms which improved included overall pain, energy level, sleep.
+ The total outlay was $500–$5000.

In his book, *Miracles Do Happen—A Physician's Experience with Alternative Medicine,* C. Norman Shealy, M.D., Ph.D., founder of the American Holistic Medical Association, and a world renowned neurosurgeon said,

"Acupuncture has been used for thousands of years in China to treat every illness imaginable. More than 300 years ago, French Jesuit priests brought the technique of acupuncture to France where it has undergone extensive scientific medical study and use. . . In 1912, Sir William Osler, the renowned medical historian, declared acupuncture to be the treatment of preference in lumbago, low back pain. . .

"I have seen miraculous instant cures of severe low back pain with a single such treatment which I've often performed since 1967. . . For both acute and chronic pain, acupuncture offers significant relief in about 80% of patients. This puts it on the par with morphine—without the risk of addiction or side effects.

" In my opinion, everyone suffering significant back pain should try acupuncture for three treatments."[2]

REFERENCES

1. Conaty, N., in *Lifeline*, the quarterly newsletter of Wisconsin Chronic Fatigue Syndrome Association, Inc.*, Winter 1999–2000, p. 9.

2. Shealy, C.N., *Miracles Do Happen—A Physician's Experience with Alternative Medicine*, Element Books, Rockport, MA, 1995, pp. 83–88.

---

*Wisconsin Cronic Fatigue Syndrome Association, Inc., 747 Lois Drive, Sun Prairie, WI 53590; www.wicfs-me.org.

Adrenal Hormones

Your two adrenal glands sit on top of each of your kidneys. They are powerful and put out hormones that are essential for life. Some you've heard about include epinephrine (Adrenalin™), cortisone, prednisolone, Medrol and other related steroid drugs. In this brief discussion, I'll focus on only two of the many, many adrenal hormones—cortisol and DHEA.

Cortisol
(hydrocortisone)

Like most professionals and nonprofessionals, I felt that cortisone and its derivatives should be used only *on* a short-term basis in people with serious—even life threatening—diseases. Then in the early 1990s, I learned about the pioneer observations of William McK. Jefferies, M.D., an endocrinologist with impeccable personal and academic credentials. In 1981 Jefferies published a book entitled *Safe Uses of Cortisone* (Charles C. Thomas publisher), and in 1994 he published a paper in which he reviewed observations he had published in peer-reviewed journals describing his success in treating people with unexplained chronic fatigue with low doses of *cortisol.* And he said,

> "When therapeutic trials of cortisol are used in patients with CFS a noticeable improvement usually occurs within a few hours after the first dose and patients often describe the return of symptoms within a few hours of a missed dose. Occasionally, improvement is not noticed until 10–14 days after treatment has begun. Patients have been treated with this schedule of cortisol or cortisone acetate for as long as 40 years without significant problems. There is . . . no reason to fear

249

that physiologic (small) doses of cortisol will produce any of the harmful side effects of pharmacological doses."[1]

In July 2000, a short time before the manuscript of this book was completed, I received an autographed copy of Dr. Jefferies' second edition of his book, which now has a different title, *Safe Uses of Cortisol*. In commenting on the new material in this book, Dr. Jefferies said,

"This little book should answer most of your questions regarding the safety and effectiveness of physiologic doses of cortisol. I suggest that you read the Preface to the second edition and the introduction to the first edition. Then Chapters 4, 7 and 10. You would also find the other chapters interesting because lowered immunity probably contributes to the development and persistence of yeast infections."

Here's an excerpt from the Preface of the second edition,

"One of the more exciting developments during the past 14 years (since the publication of the first edition of Dr. Jefferies book) has been the elucidation of the relationship between the hypothalamus, the pituitary and the adrenals (HPA axis) in response to stress and infections and in the development of autoimmune disorders. . . The rationale for prolonged use of physiologic uses of cortisol . . . makes it advisable for practicing physicians to be aware of the availability and safety of this type of therapy . . . for patients with . . . autoimmune disorders, chronic allergies and the chronic fatigue syndrome."[2]

In his book *From Fatigued to Fantastic*, Jacob Teitelbaum, M.D., said,

"If your symptoms started suddenly after a viral infection, if you're suffering from hypoglycemia, or if you have recurrent infections that take a long time to resolve, you probably have an underactive adrenal gland. About two-thirds of my severe chronic fatigue patients have an underactive or marginally functioning adrenal gland or decreased adrenal reserve."[3]

In his book, _Detoxification and Healing—The Key to Optimal Health,_ Dr. Sidney MacDonald Baker, discussed low-dose hydrocortisone therapy. Here are excerpts.

"Hydrocortisone is a normal product of your adrenal gland . . . The average daily production of hydrocortisone in your body is about 30–40 mg. If you have adrenal insufficiency (low adrenal function) you may be producing only 15–24 mg. daily. Consequently, you may feel cold and tired, have many sensitivities, low blood pressure and salt craving. By supplementing your low production with, say 5–20 mg. of hydrocortisone, your body supply becomes normal and symptoms should promptly disappear."

In his continuing discussion Baker points out that people often misunderstand this type of therapy because of their concern about the side effects from the use of high-dose cortisone-containing medications, prednisone and Medrol. And in his patients where he feels this therapy is indicated, he prescribes cortisol beginning at 2.5 mg daily and gradually working up to a maximum dose of 20 mg a day. If they show no difference in their symptoms, including feeling cold, tired and dizzy, other causes of their problems are looked for.

"This diagnostic trial is free of risk and should give an answer to the question of mild adrenal insufficiency within three weeks. . . Remember this is a low dose treatment and is very different from taking steroids in large amounts."[4] (emphasis added)

DHEA
(Dehydroepiandrosterone)

I knew nothing about DHEA until I heard a lecture by Julian Whitaker, M.D., at a conference of the American College of

Advancement in Medicine in the early 1990s. Then in the February 1994 issue of his newsletter, Whitaker said,

> "DHEA is the 'mother' hormone produced by the adrenal gland. Your body readily converts it on demand into active hormones such as estrogen and progesterone . . . In addition, DHEA decline signals age-related disease."[5]

In his continuing discussion, Whitaker cited research studies by several physicians, including Elizabeth Barrett-Connor, M.D., of the University of California School of Medicine (San Diego) and Eugene Roberts, M.D.

I learned more about DHEA from Dr. Elmer Cranton, a graduate of Harvard Medical School and my friend and consultant for over 25 years. In 1996 he published a book entitled *Resetting the Clock—5 Anti-Aging Hormones That Are Revolutionizing the Quality and Length Of Life*. Other hormones in addition to DHEA discussed in this book (which was co-authored by William Fryer) are human growth hormone (HGH), melatonin, estrogen and testosterone.

In an 18-page chapter, "DHEA: Super Hormone in Search of Its Identity," Cranton describes some of his experiences in treating his patients with DHEA during the previous five years. And he said,

> "I made careful laboratory measurements of blood levels to ensure that what I gave them brought them only up to what was normal in a healthy young adult. The response was pretty striking."

Many symptoms in these patients improved, including energy, improved sleep, thicker and moister skin, migraines, sex drive and depression. He also cited a study carried out by Samuel Yen, M.D., and colleagues at the La Jolla campus of the University of California. These researchers published a double-blind study on 13 men and 17 women between the ages of 40 and 70 who were given the "replacement" dose of DHEA. Patients in the study were given DHEA for three months and a fake pill (placebo) for another three months. None of them knew who was receiving which pill until the code was broken at the end of the study. In discussing this study Cranton said,

> "Since the 30 subjects were all healthy there was never any question of curing illness. What happened however—measured by answers to lengthy questionnaires—was startling enough. *An overwhelming majority (67% of the men and 84% of the women) reported 'a remarkable increase in perceived physical and psychological well-being' during the period in which they were on DHEA.* (emphasis added)
>
> "My own experience with patients has shown over and over how frequently they come back after taking DHEA for a while and tell me—in vague but glowing terms—that their life has somehow just improved . . . A few of the conditions . . . that have been reported improve when DHEA is administered, including allergies, Alzheimer's, arthritis, chemical sensitivities, elevated cholesterol, Epstein-Barr Syndrome, herpes, liver disorders, Lupus, menopause, recurrent infections and senility."[6]

In a comprehensive review of DHEA Alan R. Gaby, M.D., included these comments.

> "Dehydroepiandrosterone is . . . secreted in greater quantity by the adrenal gland than any other adrenal steroid . . . Circulating levels of DHEA decline progressively with age; this age-related decline does not occur with any of the other adrenal steroids. Epidemiologic evidence indicates that higher DHEA levels are associated with increased longevity and prevention of heart disease and cancer, suggesting that some of the manifestations of aging may be caused by DHEA deficiency. Animal and laboratory data indicate that administration of DHEA may prevent obesity, diabetes, cancer (breast, colon

and liver) and heart disease; enhance the functioning of the immune system; and prolong life.

"In humans, evidence exists that DHEA might be associated with autoimmune diseases such as lupus, rheumatoid arthritis and multiple sclerosis; chronic fatigue syndrome; acquired immunodeficiency syndrome (AIDS); allergic disorders; osteoporosis; and Alzheimer's disease. Although the administration of DHEA appears to be safe, its long-term effects are unknown, and it is possible that adverse consequences will become evident with chronic use. It is therefore important that this hormone be used with care and that practitioners err on the side of caution when contemplating DHEA supplementation."[7]

I found further information about DHEA in a six-page discussion on the Internet. Here are excerpts.

"Claims have appeared that DHEA is an antiaging hormone; but to date, no human research supports this claim. The fact that young people have higher levels of DHEA than older people does not necessarily mean that supplementing DHEA will make people younger. In double-blind research, DHEA has improved a sense of well-being in some, but not all, studies. . .

"Equal levels of DHEA do not appear in food, and therefore, 'dietary deficiency' does not exist. Some people, however, may not synthesize enough DHEA. DHEA levels peak in early adulthood and then start a lifelong descent. By the age of sixty, DHEA levels are only about 5–15% of what they were at their peak at younger ages.

"Most people do not need to supplement DHEA. The question of who should take this hormone remains controversial. Some experts believe the 5–15 mg of DHEA for women and 10–30 mg for men are appropriate amounts, depending on blood levels of DHEA or DHEAS. . . People should consult a nutritionally oriented doctor to have DHEA levels monitored before and during supplementation. *Only people with low blood levels of DHEA or DHEAS should take this hormone until more is known about its effects.*"[8] (emphasis added)

My Comments: DHEA seems to be an extremely useful supplement for some people with chronic health disorders including those who are tired. And based on the study by Dr. Yen and colleagues at the University of California, it may help others who appear to be healthy. *I feel that its administration should be supervised by a health professional experienced in its use.* If you do not have such a professional and want to take the hormone, read *Resetting the Clock* by Elmer Cranton, M.D. (co-authored by William Fryer). You can order this book by calling 800-337-9918. In this book you'll find instructions on when and how much DHEA to take, as well as cautions, side effects and drug interactions.

You may also find other publications in your health food store, including *DHEA—The Youth and Health Hormone* by Norman Shealy, M.D., and *DHEA—A Practical Guide* by Ray Sahelian, M.D. You can also get a list of DHEA references by sending a long, self-addressed, stamped envelope to Phillips Publishing Company, Service-DHEA, 7811 Monroe Rd., Potomac, MD 20854.

REFERENCES

1. Jefferies, W. McK., *Safe Uses of Cortisone,* Charles C. Thomas, Springfield, 1981 and Jefferies, W.M., "Mild Adreno-Cortico Deficiency; Chronic Allergies, Autoimmune Disorders and the Chronic Fatigue Syndrome: A continuation of the cortisone story," *Medical Hypotheses,* 1994; 42:183–189.

2. Jefferies, W.McK., *Safe Uses of Cortisol,* Second edition, Charles C. Thomas, Springfield, 1996, p. vi.

3. Teitelbaum, J., *From Fatigued to Fantastic,* Avery Publishing Co., New York, 1986, p. 31.

4. Baker, S.M., *Detoxification and Healing—The Key to Optimal Health,* Keats Publishing, Inc., New Canaan, CT, 1997, pp. 133–137.

5. Whitaker, J., *Health and Healing—Tomorrow's Medicine Today*, Phillips Publishing, Inc., Potomac, MD.

6. Cranton, E., *Resetting the Clock—5 Anti-Aging Hormones That Are Revolutionizing the Quality and Length Of Life*, M. Evans and Company, New York, 1996.

7. Gaby, A.R., "Dehydroepiandrosterone: Biological Effects and Clinical Significance," *Alternative Medicine Review*, Vol. 1 No 2, 1996.

8. www.puritan.com/healthnotes

Airborne Allergens and Fatigue

Although most of my attention as an allergist focused on food allergies and sensitivities as a cause of fatigue, headache and other nervous symptoms, similar symptoms can be caused by inhaled allergens. A dramatic case report I remember reading some 40 years ago was that of a California physician who became tired and depressed each spring. His wife and his professional associates said in effect, "Joe must become exhausted because he works so hard through the winter. And his fatigue is psychological because when he takes off for a vacation his tired feelings disappear."

Then an allergist did detective work which included testing Joe for pollens. And to his delight, he found the answer. Joe was sensitive to the tree pollens in his yard and neighborhood. Following immunotherapy he was able to work through the springtime pollen season without developing fatigue and take his vacation with his family during the summer when his children were out of school.

During a visit to my office one day, one of my adult patients with food and chemical sensitivities and yeast-related problems said, "I've just returned from visiting my daughter and my grandchild. They live in an old house that smells musty and moldy. Almost from the moment that I set foot in the door, I began to 'feel funny.' Although my nose became stuffy, my worst symptoms were feeling tired and in a fog. These symptoms worsened the longer I stayed in my daughter's home. When I returned to my home and breathed fresh air, my symptoms began to subside.

I told my daughter, "When I come back for our next visit, we'll get together at my motel or anywhere but your beautiful old home."

In his book *Tired All the Time*,[1] Dr. Ronald Hoffman told the story of a 22-year-old woman who was suffering from extraordinary fatigue, headaches, jitteriness and inability to concentrate. When her physician could not find a physical cause for her symptoms, he referred her to a psychologist who concluded that she was having a severe emotional problem.

Then, she went to see Dr. Hoffman who took her history and learned that her symptoms developed when she moved to a new building. So he instantly suspected that she was suffering from the "sick building syndrome." He asked her to take mold plates to her office and expose them. When the mold plates were returned and analyzed they showed a total fungus and mold growth too numerous to count. The woman's employer hired a firm to clean the ducts in the building's cooling system and her fatigue and other symptoms disappeared.

Molds are more apt to multiply where there's dampness and many different molds can cause symptoms, including *hormodendrum, alternaria* and *aspergillus*. How do you find out which molds are causing problems? I first found the answer to this question from Dr. Sherry Rogers who published three studies in the *Annals of Allergy* in the early 1980s[2, 3]. In her studies, Dr. Rogers assessed the 24-hour environment of her patients for 13 months. At a conference of the American Academy of Environmental Medicine Dr. Rogers presented her findings; here are some of the points she emphasized.

Immunotherapy with yeast and mold extracts often help, but they may not help as much as we would like. When such therapy is not effective, it may be because the mold extracts used do not accurately represent the fungi bothering the patient.

In another study she found that with a better gel or agar in the mold plates a physician could find 30% more molds which could cause symptoms.

To more accurately obtain proper yeast and mold extracts for testing and treatment often requires cultures of the patient's home or office. Dr. Rogers discusses the role molds play in making people sick in her many books, including *Tired or Toxic?* and *Depression—Cured At Last.* Physicians can obtain information about culturing molds and Dr. Rogers by writing to Mold Survey Service, 2800 W. Genessee St., Syracuse, NY 13219 or by calling 800-846-6687.*

In July 2000, Dr. Rogers sent me further comments about her observations and publications. Here are excerpts.

> "I've seen many chronically ill patients who have been told, 'There's no known cause or cure for your problems.' By giving these patients special mold allergy injections, problems including fatigue, weakness, dizziness, asthma, migraines, total body eczema and other symptoms cleared. I described some of my observations in an article published over a decade ago. I've also discussed these observations in my book *No More Heartburn*. Included in this book is a discussion of many new over-the-counter yeast fighters."[4]

The cover story of the August 18–20, 2000 issue of *USA Weekend* was entitled, "Mold in Schools: a health alert," by Arnold Mann. This article told how molds in schools were making children sick. Symptoms caused by molds included asthma, sinus infections, headaches, coughing and eye and throat irritations. The mold problem was so bad that a Texas city (El Paso) has spent $4.2 million for mold renovations in 14 schools.

---

*You can obtain additional information about Dr. Rogers' books and other publications from Prestige Publishing, P.O. Box 3068, Syracuse, NY 13220. Phone: 800-846-6687. Web page: www.prestigepublishing.com.

According to the article, some molds may "produce airborne toxins called mycotoxins, which can cause even more serious problems, including chronic fatigue, loss of balance and memory, irritability and difficulty speaking."*

REFERENCES

1. Hoffman, R., *Tired All the Time,* Poseidon Press, New York, 1993, pp. 132–133.

2. Terraria, F., Rogers, S.A., "In-home Fungal Studies: Methods to increase the yield," *Annals of Allergy,* 49:35–37, July 1983.

3. Rogers, S.A., "A 13-month work, leisure, sleep, environmental fungal survey," *Annals of Allergy,* 52:338–341, May 1984.

4. Rogers, S.A., "Resistant Cases: Response to mold immunotherapy and environmental and dietary controls," *Clinical Ecology,* 5,3:115–120, 1987/1988.

*More information about how to spot and treat mold-related respiratory problems can be obtained from the American Lung Association, 1-800-lungusa (586-4872).

Dental Fillings

If your CFS is yeast-connected, you'll nearly always improve when you change your diet, clean up your home environment, take prescription and nonprescription antifungal agents, avoid foods that cause sensitivity reactions, take probiotics and other nutritional supplements.

But, if you have CFS and you are doing all these things and are at a standstill, it could be because you are absorbing toxins from the mercury/silver amalgam fillings in your mouth.*

The hazards of silver-mercury fillings have been talked about by a handful of dentists during the past decade. According to those who oppose the use of these fillings, they can cause toxic reactions and play a part in making people sick. Symptoms attributed to these fillings include fatigue, headache, central nervous system dysfunction, muscle and joint pains and disturbances in other parts of the body.

This controversy was discussed on CBS's *60 Minutes* in the early 1990s. On this program, Dr. Murray J. Vimy of the University of Calgary Medical School and Alfred Zamm, M.D., of Kingston, New York, presented information on the potential and actual toxic effects of mercury-amalgam fillings. Vimy had placed silver fillings in the mouths of pregnant sheep. Three days later, mercury was found in the blood of mothers and fetuses and in the amniotic fluid. Two weeks later, it was found in other tissue samples.

---

*Dentists who would like a free packet of information on proper protocol for safe amalgam removal can write to Grant H. Layton, D.D.S., 16905 Avenida De Acacias, Box 2184, Rancho Santa Fe, CA 92067. eda1@ix.netcom.com

In April 1991, I attended a seminar in San Diego, California, sponsored by the Environmental Dental Association. During this seminar, the then president of EDA, Joyal Taylor, D.D.S., gave a demonstration that impressed me.

Volunteers from the audience were tested with a special probe which measured the release of mercury vapor following chewing. One of the volunteers had no fillings in her mouth and the second had a number of fillings. (The machine for testing mercury vapors is used in submarines by the U.S. Navy, as well as the Environmental Protection Agency, EPA.) The woman with dental fillings showed a high level of mercury, while the other woman showed none.

You may wish to consider the removal of your silver-mercury fillings if your chronic health problems haven't improved in spite of your efforts, and those of your physicians. Based on the observations I've obtained for the past several years, *the possibility of dental mercury toxicity should be investigated by a dentist familiar with the problem.*

Further information, including a list of mercury-free dentists in your area, can be obtained from the Environmental Dental Association (EDA), 800-388-8124. Mercury-free dental fillings are also discussed in the Holistic Dental Digest by Jerry Mittelman, D.D.S. For a sample copy of his newsletter, send a long SASE to Dr. Mittelman, 263 West End, #2A, New York, NY 10023.

Books that provide information on mercury/amalgam dental fillings include:

+ *The Complete Guide to Mercury Toxicity from Dental Fillings,* Joyal Taylor, D.D.S., available from the Environmental Dental Association, P.O. Box 2184, Rancho Santa Fe, CA 92067. $14.95 plus $3.00 shipping.

+ *Are Your Dental Fillings Poisoning You?*, Guy S. Fasciana, D.M.D., Keats Publishing Co., 27 Pine St., New Canaan, CT 06840.
+ *The Toxic Time Bomb*, Sam Ziff, D.D.S., 4401 Real Court, Orlando, FL 32808.

Electroacupuncture and Muscle Testing

n the mid 1980s, a physician interested in yeast-related problems told me about an instrument he had obtained from Germany designed by Dr. Reinhold Voll. During a visit to his office I saw him put an electronic probe on various parts of a patient's hands. He told me that with this instrument he was able to determine the foods his patient was sensitive to and the therapies he would use in treating him. Although I did my best to pay attention to his demonstration, I did not understand the technique and why or how it would work. To summarize, it didn't interest me.

Several years later, along with a half dozen other physicians interested in food allergies/sensitivities and yeast problems, I visited the office of James O'Shea, a board-certified pediatrician who received part of his training at the Massachusetts General Hospital. During our mini conference, Dr. O'Shea demonstrated a special filter which removed chemicals from tap water. He also showed us how he carried out serial dilution testing to determine the proper dose of allergy extracts.

Then he had one of his patients demonstrate muscle testing. In carrying out this testing, an object (such as an apple) was put in the person's hand. Or the person would drink a sip of milk and hold it in their mouth. The person being tested would then hold her arm out at a right angle while the technician administering the test would apply pressure to push the arm down.

If the apple, milk (or whatever substance being tested) disagreed, the arm could be pushed down with only a minimal amount of pressure. By contrast, if the substance caused no problem, the person being tested could resist the pressure and the arm would remain extended. Using the same muscle testing technique he also showed how he could determine the strength of an allergy extract to use in treating a patient with pollen, mold and dust mite allergy. Although I was amazed, I did not pursue this method of testing in my own practice.

A few months later, my good friend Elmer Cranton, M.D., who at that time was living and working in a small community in southwest Virginia, told me about muscle testing. He said that a patient (a woman with a Ph.D. degree and member of the faculty of a neighboring university) had found that muscle testing was an effective way to identify the foods that were causing her problems.

During the decade of the 1990s, other people, including both professionals and nonprofessionals, told me that muscle testing and electroacupuncture provided them with valuable diagnostic and therapeutic information. I did not discuss either of these techniques in my lectures or books because I said to myself,

> "I'm already involved in writing and talking about other controversial subjects, including food and chemical sensitivities and yeast-related problems. Although these methods of testing and treating people seem to have merit, they would be even more controversial than 'the yeast connection.' And gaining credibility and acceptance for the yeast hypothesis is my main mission."

While gathering material for *Tired—So Tired!*, I called and wrote to many knowledgeable and experienced professionals. Questions I asked included, "Which prescription and nonprescription antifungal agents have you found to be most effective?" One of the professionals, Susanna Choi, M.D., a board-certified

Colorado gynecologist, rather than discussing antifungal medications said,

> "I'm very excited about electroacupuncture testing and diagnosis. Call our mutual friend, Dr. Kathy Gibbons, and she'll tell you more about it."

So I called Kathy on July 18, 2000, and with her permission I recorded our conversation. Here are excerpts.

WGC: Kathy, when did you first become interested in electroacupuncture testing?

KG: Last fall, when I was working with Dr. Choi, we had three or four patients who came into the office and said "please write a prescription" for a particular product. When we asked why, each said *"the machine says I need it."* So after hearing this request several times, Dr. Choi came in to me and said, "Kathy, what is this machine?" So we started looking into electroacupuncture and meridian stress testing.

We had the salesman come in and demonstrate his equipment. Before he came in, Dr. Choi and I were convinced we were not going to buy the machine, and the meeting with him would convince us not to buy it. However, we were really surprised. We came out of the demonstration meeting, where he tested both of us, saying, "We have to buy it." *The instrument gave a correct test result for every substance we tested, and the salesman knew nothing about us ahead of time.*

WGC: It can test not only for foods you're sensitive to, but also for hormones and medications?

KG: Yes. The instrument can be used to see if progesterone is needed, and to see which type of progesterone is best tolerated. It can also be used to see if other hormones are needed, such as testosterone. The instrument is not approved by the FDA as a diagnostic tool, but it sure helps guide you along as to what a patient needs. Of course you would back the instrument up with blood work.

For example, we found people whose thyroid meridian was really stressed according to the instrument. So based on that we did blood work on those patients. And 70 to 80% of the time we picked up thyroid problems. We would not have normally done blood work on those types of patients, and so those are thyroid problems that we would have missed.

WGC: Amazing—almost unbelievable. Kathy tell me again about your credentials—I know they're impressive.

KG: I received my Ph.D. in biochemistry from the University of Illinois. I've worked in nutritional counseling for ten years, and, as you know, I worked for Dr. Choi for the last five years. Just two months ago I decided to set up my own office so that I could use the instrument on all family members, not just the OB/GYN patients that Dr. Choi treats. The instrument is just so powerful that I wanted to be able to use it for anyone.

WGC: Kathy, I'm excited about what you're telling me. Does testing with this instrument tell you whether or not you need more magnesium, or more B_1 or more B_6?

KG: The instrument will definitely indicate whether or not magnesium, for example, will reduce stress on the body. The same is true for B_1, B_6 or any other vitamin or supplement. You can use the instrument to stress test on magnesium, and the instrument will tell you if your magnesium level is off. It won't tell you whether the level is too high or too low. It'll do the same thing for your vitamins and minerals. Once the instrument tells you there's something wrong, you can figure out by doing various other tests whether you have been taking too much or too little. You can also test amino acids, digestive aids, vaccines, and essential fatty acids—there are just so many ways you can use it.

What I do when I first test a patient is to do a baseline and then a nutritional analysis. I go into all the libraries of data stored in the instrument and determine what is out of balance. Many times you'll find all the vitamins are fine but the minerals are really out of balance, or the essential fatty acids are really off. Once I've determined that, I go back and decide if that

267

person has too much or too little of each vitamin or other supplement, and then I start coming up with a nutritional program for them that incorporates what I've learned.

Electroacupuncture testing also helps me to evaluate allergies to inhalants and chemicals. Using it I found that one of our chronically ill patients was sensitive to chlorine.

The person doing the testing must be knowledgeable, skilled and experienced. You have to know what you're doing. You have to know what you're looking for and you have to go look for it. What you're able to do is just look "all over the place" so much more quickly than ever before.

Here's one example. Maybe you wonder if the patient has parasites. The electro testing helps provide you with a clue. That doesn't mean you don't need to run the Great Smokies Lab stool tests to identify the parasites. You do need to do those tests. But the instrument gives you a really quick way of searching to find out which directions you should go and what would make the most sense.

The instrument I use is made by BioMeridian, a Salt Lake City company that combined the technologies from several smaller companies and put them together. I did not check into instruments made in Europe.

WGC: What does the Colorado Medical Society say about this kind of testing?

KG: The instrument is an FDA-approved instrument, and from what I understand it meets all of the new guidelines for the most recent FDA certification level. But it is not approved for diagnostic work. So if you pick up that someone has a stressed thyroid, you need to run the conventional medical tests before prescribing thyroid. The key is this–the instrument just gets you so much quicker to the right treatment for a patient. That's why I'm so excited about it.

WGC: A final thing. How about your patients with a yeast-related problem? Does it help you tell whether Diflucan or Sporanox is the way to go?

KG: Definitely. You can stress test on candida. In fact, I have a library of about 22 yeast-related organisms and we can stress test on all of those very quickly. Then you can test a drug or herbal remedy and see which one works best for that patient.

My Comments: Because of the personal and academic credentials of Dr. Choi and Dr. Gibbons, two friends I've met and visited with during trips to Colorado, I am impressed with the validity of electroacupuncture and muscle testing.

If you call or write me and say, "Dr. Crook, should I go to a health professional who uses these machines?" I would repeat and expand on the comments of Dr. Gibbons who said, "The person doing the testing must be knowledgeable, skilled and experienced."

I'd also say, "Check on the person's credentials and reputation in your community. Find out if the professional is kind and caring and professionally competent in caring for patients. Also get an idea about what her/his services will cost and whether you feel comfortable with her/his ability to provide you with continuing care." Still another question, "Would he/she provide you with the results of your test findings so that you can share them with your own personal physician?"

A final comment. Whether it's for electroacupuncture testing or any type of diagnostic studies or therapy, your goal is to find a health professional who exemplifies these qualities: COMPE-TENCE, UNSELFISHNESS, KINDNESS and CARING.

Gastrointestinal Support Program

The goal of this therapeutic program is to "support the improvement . . . of the various GI functions through appropriate evaluation, indicated therapy, nutritional, digestive enzyme, pre-and probiotics support."

Here are some of the things I learned from a six-page discussion of Dr. Jeffrey Bland's 4R™ Program*.

The first R, *remove,* refers to the elimination of any pathogenic microflora and/or parasites that may be present. In discussing the therapies that may be necessary, Bland pointed out that simply "adding probiotics, nutrients or digestive enzymes will not usually be enough." He also emphasized the importance of removing foods from the diet which cause allergic/sensitivity reactions, especially dairy and gluten-containing grains and cereal foods.

In discussing the second R, *replace,* Bland said that it refers to the replacement of digestive factors and/or enzymes whose intrinsic, functional secretion may be limited or inadequate. He also said that there were other factors, including hydrochloric acid, intrinsic factor, bile and a number of enzymes.

Bland said that the third R, *reinoculate,* refers to the introduction of two commonly used and "well researched genera of mi-

---

*Condensed and adapted from TECHNICAL BULLETIN—REMOVE, REPLACE, REINOCULATE, REPAIR. THE 4R™ GASTROINTESTINAL SUPPORT PROGRAM, HealthComm, International Inc., P.O. Box 1729, 5800 Soundview Dr., Gig Harbor, WA 98335, USA. Phone: 253-851-3943. Fax: 253-851-9749. www.healthcomm.com.

croflora," _lactobacillus_ and _bifidobacteria_. He pointed out that these substances are available as oral supplements in the form of powders, tablets and capsules and that they should be kept at cool temperatures and product lifetime dates should be considered.

In discussing the fourth R, _repair,_ Bland said that it "refers to providing nutritional support for regeneration or healing of the gastrointestinal mucosa." In his discussion he said that the lactulose/mannitol permeability tests may be useful in assessing individuals with chronic health problems. Many different nutrients are needed which he said were "critical" in intestinal cell wall structure and function. Among those he listed were antioxidants, vitamins and minerals.

In discussing this program Bland said that when considered together, the four steps of the 4R™ gastrointestinal support program appropriately address, from a clinical standpoint, underlying dysfunction. "In evaluating any individual's health and nutritional status, each of the above factors can contribute to increasing and self-generating pathophysiology."

Light

I first learned about the importance of *broad spectrum* light over 20 years ago. At that time I saw a movie and read reports by Dr. John Ott of Sarasota, Florida. While working with Walt Disney he learned that pumpkin seed sprouts would not fully mature under the ordinary fluorescent light and flourished when ultraviolet light was added.

In the 1970s, Ott and colleagues studied 104 first grade children. In classrooms with ordinary cool white fluorescent lights, some students demonstrated hyperactivity, fatigue, irritability and attentional deficits. *In classrooms with full spectrum lighting classroom performance improved remarkably one month after the new lights were installed.*

Based on Ott's research studies, the Duro-Test Corporation began using the full spectrum fluorescent tubes of Vita-Lite and installed them in my office.

How does good, natural, full spectrum light work and what can it do for you? It favorably influences your immune system, your hormones, the formation of vitamin D, the absorption of calcium and phosphorus, your ability to pay attention and much more.

To obtain the health benefits of light you should spend at least a half hour a day outdoors in natural light and/or obtain special broad spectrum lights for your home and office. These lights, which fit into standard fluorescent fixtures, can be purchased in garden supply stores, hardware stores, some lighting departments and health food stores.

Seasonal Affective Disorder (SAD): This disorder is characterized by fatigue and depression that occurs about the same time each year. It comes on in the winter and goes away in the spring. It especially affects people who live in the northern part of the U.S. and Canada as compared to those who live in Florida and other southern states where people spend more time outdoors during winter months.

According to Jacob Liberman, O.D., Ph.D., in his book _LIGHT—Medicine of the Future_,[1]

> "This condition, found more often in women than in men (4 to 1) usually is accompanied by overeating, excessive sleeping, weight gain, reduced sex drive and sometimes lowering of immune function. SAD is thought to arise in part from high levels of melatonin brought on by the shortened day length and less available daylight associated with winter.
>
> "Although the exact mechanism of the reaction is unknown, bright light treatment by way of the eyes has been found to have significant antidepressant effect on more than 80% of those suffering from SAD or its milder form called 'winter blues.'"

Dr. Liberman also cited the research studies carried out by Dr. Fritz Hollwich. Here's an excerpt.

> "In 1980 Dr. Fritz Hollwich conducted a study comparing the effects of sitting under strong artificial cool white illumination, versus the effects of sitting under strong artificial light that simulates sunlight. Using changes in the endocrine system to evaluate the effects, he found stress-like levels of ACTH and cortisol in individuals sitting under the cool white tubes. These changes were totally absent in the individual sitting under the sunlight stimulating tubes. . .Hollwich's findings clarify and substantiate the observations of Ott and others regarding the agitated physical behavior, fatigue and reduced mental capacities of children spending their entire days at school under artificial illumination."

He also cites the work of Dr. Darell Boyd Harmon which began in 1938 when the Texas Department of Health initiated a long-range comprehensive program with child development. When changes were instituted at a Texas school in 1946, there were percentage reductions in several of the children's problem areas, including visual difficulties (65%), nutritional problems (47.8%) and fatigue (55.6%).

"In addition to these apparent improvements in physical well being, some comparable results were also seen in academic achievement, even though no attempt was made in any of the centers to study or augment curriculum education philosophy of methodology."

My Comments: *If you're "sick and tired" make sure that your treatment program includes adequate amounts of "good light."*

REFERENCES

1. Liberman, Jacob, O.D., Ph.D., *Light—Medicine of the Future*, Beare & Company Publishing, Santa Fe, NM, 1991. Dr. Liberman's address: Universal Light Technology, P.O. Box 520, Carbondale, CO 81623. 303-927-0100.

Magnets

I first began hearing about magnets about ten years ago. At that time, William H. Philpott, M.D., an Oklahoma physician, sent me a lot of information about the value of magnets in treating people with health problems of many types. These included people with pain, sleep problems, respiratory disorders, digestive problems and much more. I met Dr. Philpott several years ago and had dinner with him and I knew he was a creative, innovative physician. Although I read the material he sent me, I didn't get really interested in the subject.

In the next several years a number of people who wrote to me told me that magnets had helped them. Included was a friend and professional consultant who told me that a Nikken magnetic mattress helped relieve her arthritic pains.

Then almost two years ago I developed pain in my left upper leg and back. At times the pain was severe and kept me awake. Different therapies, including a back operation, provided little relief. Then my sister, Nancy Cheek, called me from Nashville and said, "Vanderbilt University has established a pain clinic. A friend of mine with pain like yours gained wonderful relief from magnets they stuck on his hip and back."

So I went to the Vanderbilt Pain Clinic and a kind, caring physician, W. Bradley Worthington, M.D., and his staff, spent two hours with me. They put seven patented "polarized" Holcomb magnets on my back and hip. They helped tremendously. Very soon 98% of my pain went away. I only stick the magnets on occasionally at night if I feel a tender spot.

In August 2000 I received a brochure from the Vanderbilt University School of Nursing announcing a seminar on Magna

Bloc™ therapy scheduled for January 20, 2001, on pain management. Included in the presentations will be a discussion of Magna Bloc™ therapy by Robert Holcomb, M.D., Ph.D. For more information you can write to Vanderbilt University School of Nursing, Magna Bloc™ Pain Management Clinic, 461 21st Ave., So., Nashville, TN 37240. 615-322-2783; Fax: 615-383-3998; e-mail: sharon.aucoin@mcmail.vanderbilt.edu.

Nuts

I love nuts and I've recommended them to my patients and my readers for many years. For example, in my 1986 book *The Yeast Connection* I said that I recommended nuts, especially freshly shelled nuts. And I cited the observations of the late Henry Schroeder, M.D., of Dartmouth College, a recognized authority on trace minerals who said,

> "Nuts . . . contain adequate or surplus amounts of all the trace elements; Coming from seeds, they contain the elements needed for the growth of the seed until the plant forms roots. . . The essential trace elements are much more important than the vitamins. They cannot be synthesized, as can vitamins . . . Without them, life would cease to exist."[1]

In *The Yeast Connection Cookbook,* my co-author Marjorie Hurt Jones, in discussing nut and seed butters said,

> "I find that the blender does a better job with nut and seed butters than a food processor. While doing the job yourself the variety is limited only to the kinds of nuts and seeds you can find."

She recommended grinding up nuts into a fine meal and then adding oil. Marge also provided readers with instructions for making nut milk and she said,

> "Quick and easy to whip up, you'll find many ways to use this creamy liquid over cereal, or in making sauces, soups, shakes, etc. . . Even though the nuts bring a fair amount of fat to the nut milk, you can adjust the amount of fat by varying the quantity of nuts."[2]

In an e-mail message to me in August 2000, Marge said,

> "One last thought about nuts. Rancidity can be a problem. I suggest buying nuts from a source where there seems to be a good turnover. Better yet, buy from a health food store that refrigerates nuts—and has a good turnover.
>
> "At home store nuts tightly sealed in the refrigerator or freezer. Purchase small quantities more often. Even though the published studies cited peanuts and almonds, nutritionally it just makes good sense to include a variety of nuts. They probably all have something beneficial going for them which is bound to vary from one species of nut to another. . . which we're only just learning about."

Comments by Jean Carper:

In her Eat Smart article which appears regularly in *USA Weekend,* in an article entitled, "Nuts, Your Super Food," Carper said,

> "If you're on a high protein, high fat, low carbohydrate diet, like the Atkins or Sugar Busters programs, you may be losing weight, but getting an overload of fatty meat and dairy food bad for overall health. Another solution. Nuts. They're packed with protein and fat that fill you up without endangering your health."[3]

Carper told readers to replace other high fat foods with nuts because they "satisfy the craving for fat." She also pointed out that based on a number of studies in the 1990s that nut eaters have less heart disease. Included was a 1992 study at Loma Linda University and an Iowa Womens' Health study.

She quotes Gene Spiller, Ph.D., director of the Health Research and Studies Center in Los Altos, California, and author of a book entitled *Healthy Nuts* (Avery), who said that contrary to public opinion nuts don't make you fat. Spiller cited a study at Brigham and Women's Hospital which found that high-fat nut eaters had lost nine pounds, while low-fat dieters gained more than six pounds. The reason according to Spiller, "Nuts curb hunger by satisfying the desire for some fat."

Comments of Beatrice Trum Hunter

In her article, "High-Fat Foods for Health?" in *Consumers' Research,* June 1999, Hunter* said that people who eat nuts regularly experience significantly less heart disease and heart fatalities than those who rarely eat them. She said that nuts are also useful in weight reduction.

She said in an 18-month study of overweight people, mostly female "hard core" dieters failed repeatedly in weight-reduction regimens. Those that were given a diet which included nuts, olives and nut oils lost 5–30 pounds and after six months, 62% of them on a high monosaturated diet continued to comply and improve, as compared to only 40% on the traditional low fat diet.

In responding to a question from a reader who wanted to buy nuts in shells and crack them as she used them, Hunter recommended these two sources: "The Carolina Cracker, P.O. Box 374, Garner, NC 27529 and Krakanut, produced by Felko Products Inc., P.O. Box 62098, St. Louis Park, MN 55426."[4]

---

*Hunter is the author of a number of books concerning food topics of importance to consumers. The most recent ones include *The Great Nutrition Robbery, The Mirage of Safety* and *The Sugar Trap and How to Avoid It.* You may send your questions about food to Beatrice Trum Hunter, c/o Consumers' Research, 800 Maryland Ave., N.E., Washington, DC 20002. For a personal reply enclose a self-addressed stamped envelope.

REFERENCES

1. Schroeder, H., M.D., *The Poisons Around Us,* Bloomington, IN, University of Bloomington, Indiana University Press, 1974, pp. 118–119.

2. Crook, W.G., and Jones, M.H., *The Yeast Connection Cookbook,* Professional Books, Jackson, TN, 1989/1997, pp. 319–321.

3. Carper, Jean, *USA Weekend,* June 23–25, 2000, p. 4.

4. Hunter, B.T., "High-Fat Foods for Health?" *Consumers' Research,* June 1999.

Organic Foods

Organic foods are foods grown on farms that do not use chemicals on the soil, on the plants or on the harvested products. Why do I recommend such foods? I'm deeply concerned about the pesticides. As you've read in my discussion of chemicals in Sections III and IV, pesticides make millions of people sick.

In a 20-page discussion of organic foods in his 1999 book, *The Staying Healthy Shopper's Guide,** Elson M. Haas, M.D., said that for the last 20 years the U.S. Agriculture industry has used more than 1 billion pounds of pesticides annually. On a more hopeful note he said,

> "The organic farming sector has grown from a modest enterprise made up of small farming networks with gross sales of $78 million in 1980 to an agricultural industry with sales of more than $4 billion in 1997. This industry has grown nearly 50% every year for the past seven years. Three out of every ten consumers are now buying organically grown produce."

Also, in an interview of general consumers by *Prevention* magazine, over 50% stated they would purchase organic foods if there were a national standard. Haas describes in detail the "Essentials of Organic Growing" and the five "Health Benefits of Organic Foods." He also lists 25 important foods which you should buy organically grown if possible. In discussing cost and availability, he said,

---

*This book is available in health food stores and bookstores or can be ordered by calling 800-841-2665.

"The cost of organic products is often higher than the same nonorganic fruit, vegetable, or grain because of the smaller size of the average farm and the additional labor involved. . . *In recent years, organic foods have become more plentiful and of higher quality and some are now available at a lower cost. More and more shoppers are finding that the taste and the reassurance of quality nutrition and chemical avoidance make buying organic worthwhile.* (emphasis added.)

"Many supermarkets offer a choice between nonorganic and organic, so consumers have an ongoing opportunity to see and taste the difference. Mail order catalogs (many found on the Internet) also provide a way to make organic food and other products accessible to more people. This movement is clearly spreading and this suggests an important trend for the future."

Haas lists eight ways of "minimizing pesticides in your food." Here are several of them.

+ Limit use of out-of-season imported produce.
+ Wash, soak and peel conventionally grown fruits and vegetables.
+ Limit your intake of red meats and factory-farmed poultry.
+ Limit your intake of fish known to be caught from polluted waters.
+ Try emphasizing fruits and vegetables that can be peeled or those that have been found to have low residues.

Here are three of the resources listed by Dr. Haas.

+ The Organic Trade Association, Greenfield , MA. 413-774-7511. www.ota.com.

+ Committee for Sustainable Agriculture (CSA). www.csa.efc.org.
+ Environmental Working Group (EWG), Washington, DC.

Price-Pottenger Nutrition Foundation

Many years ago Weston A. Price, a brilliant pioneer California dentist, went all over the world looking at people who were consuming their native diets and others in the same community who were eating western diets. Those consuming foods grown on good soil were strong and healthy. By contrast, those who were consuming foods grown on poor soil (and loaded with sugar and white flour) had poor facial structure, irregular teeth and health problems of many kinds.

Following his travels, Dr. Price in collaboration with Francis M. Pottenger, Jr., M.D., Fellow of the American College of Physicians, established the Price-Pottenger Nutrition Foundation in 1965. This nutrition education foundation is the repository of research papers, books, articles and the collections of the work of Dr. Price. This foundation also continues to publish Dr. Price's classic book, *Nutrition and Physical Degeneration*.

About 20 years ago I met Marian Patricia (Pat) Connolly, the curator of *PPNF*. On a number of occasions since that time we've discussed nutrition and yeast-related problems.

The PPNF also publishes quarterly the *PPNF Journal*. Here are a few "tidbits" from their Spring 2000 *Health & Healing Wisdom—Millennium Issue*.

Peas: *If you eat peas fresh from your garden you get 100% of the vitamins present in the pea.* If you buy canned peas at the supermarket, here's what happens: 30% of the vitamins are lost in the cooking at the canning plants; 25% are lost during sterilization; 27% float away in the discarded liquid; 12% are lost when you re-heat the peas out of the can. You end up with peas that have lost 90% of the vitamins they started out with. Frozen peas are an improvement. They lose a mere 83% of their vitamins during processing.

Pesticides: A report published in the prestigious medical journal *The Lancet* (December 18, 1999) suggests a link between exposure to organochlorine compounds which have been used in pesticides and cancer of the pancreas. They also found that patients with high concentrations of DDT and three major PCBs were over five times more likely to have a mutation of the pancreatic cancer gene than patients with low levels. More information is available on the Internet at www.thelancet.com.

If you're interested in truly good nutrition and related topics, you may wish to join PPNF. You can obtain more information by calling 1-800-366-3748 or sending an e-mail message to info@price-pottenger.org. Or you can send a fax to PPNF, P.O. Box 2614, La Mesa, CA 91943-2164. Fax: 619-574-1314.

Sleep

In the early 1990s I began to hear about melatonin. So did millions of other people who saw it in their health food stores. A number of books were also written about this hormone which helped people sleep, but also strengthened the immune system.

In his 1996 book (co-authored by William Fryer), my friend Elmer Cranton devoted two chapters to melatonin, including one entitled "Melatonin: Sleep King." He said,

> "Melatonin's capacity to aid in sleep enhancement is not disputed by even the most skeptical critics of this hormone's new-found celebrity. . . The amount you should take will, therefore, vary quite naturally according to your age. My recommendation is that from age 45 to 54, take 0.2 to 1 mg. . . But if you find a slightly larger dose produces more benefit, there's no evidence it will harm you."[1]

Many people with CFS, fibromyalgia and related disorders experience trouble sleeping and physicians have used a number of different prescription medications in helping them, including a group of drugs called benzodiazepines (Ativan, Halcion, Librium, Xanax, Serax). Although these drugs help, prolonged use is not recommended by most physicians because individuals who take them on a regular basis may become dependent.

A 1999 study shows that melatonin may provide an answer for people with CFS and fibromyalgia. In this study, researchers from Israel described their observations. Here's a summary.

> "Thirty-four subjects receiving benzodiazepine therapy were enrolled in the 2-period study. In period 1, patients re-

ceived (double-blinded) melatonin (2 mg in a controlled-release formulation) or a placebo nightly for 6 weeks. They were encouraged to reduce their benzodiazepine 50% during week 2, 75% during weeks 3 and 4, and to discontinue benzodiazepine therapy completely during weeks 5 and 6.

"In period 2, melatonin was administered (single-blinded) for 6 weeks to all subjects and attempts to discontinue benzodiazepine therapy were resumed. Benzodiazepine consumption and subjective sleep-quality scores were reported daily by all patients. All subjects were then allowed to continue melatonin therapy and follow-up reassessments were performed 6 months later."

Here's a summary of their results:

+ 14 of the 18 subjects who had received melatonin were able to discontinue benzodiazepine therapy. By contrast, only 4 of the 16 in the placebo group were able to do so. (P = .006).
+ Those who received melatonin therapy showed significantly higher "sleep-quality" scores. (P = .04).
+ Six additional subjects in the placebo group were able to stop benzodiazepine therapy when given melatonin in period 2.
+ A 6-month follow-up of these patients showed that of the 24 patients who stopped taking benzodiazepine and received melatonin therapy, 19 maintained good sleep quality.

The authors concluded from their study that,

"Controlled-release melatonin may effectively facilitate discontinuation of benzodiazepine therapy while maintaining good sleep quality."[2]

An editorial accompanying this report discussed the various aspects of this study. In the concluding sentence of this editorial, Harold H. Bursztajn said,

". . . Clinicians have the opportunity and health care organizations have the responsibility to facilitate making available as a choice effective benzodiazepine-free treatment for insomnia. Choosing benzodiazepine-free treatment for insomnia can help patients sleep, dream, remember, and continue to have access to both the continuity of autobiographical memories relevant to authenticity and the procedural memory essential to autonomy."[3]

REFERENCES

1. Cranton, E. and Fryer, W., *Resetting the Clock,* M. Evans, New York, NY, 1996, pp. 136–142.

2. Garfunkel, D., et al., "Facilitation of benzodiazepine discontinuation by melatonin: a new clinical approach," *Archives of Internal Medicine,* November 8, 1999, 159(20):2456–60. Can be found on the Internet at www.ncbi.nlm.nih.gov.

3. Bursztajn, H.J., "Melatonin Therapy: From Benzodiazepine-Dependent Insomnia to Authenticity and Autonomy," *Archives of Internal Medicine,* November 8, 1999, 159(20):2393–95.

Tests

In all of my books that deal with yeast-connected health problems, I emphasize the importance of a person's history. I've found that by using my Candida Questionnaire and Score Sheet a person can usually determine whether their health problems are yeast related.[1]

Many individuals with fatigue, headache, depression, digestive problems, muscle and joint aches have taken numerous tests which have not helped them. Here's an example of what I'm talking about. In a letter to me, 40-year-old Amy said,

> "I've spent thousands of dollars on tests of all kinds—x-rays, blood tests, MRIs and much more. Every opening in my body has been looked into. After reviewing these tests, my physicians have said, 'We can't find anything *really wrong* with you.'"

Does this mean that tests do not help? My answer is "No."

In a chapter "Testing: The Key to Understanding the Causes of Your Chronic Fatigue," in the book *Alternative Medicine Guide to Chronic Fatigue, Fibromyalgia and Environmental Illness,*[2] the authors listed the following tests: electrodermal screening, anti-candida antibodies panel, stool analysis, CBC blood test report, immune system testing, hormone testing, heavy metal toxicity screening, testing for enzyme deficiencies, allergy testing and testing for nutritional deficiencies.

Some of these tests may help when ordered and interpreted by a professional skilled in their use. Of those listed, I've been especially impressed with the value of the Comprehensive Digestive Stool Analysis (CDSA). This test is especially useful in identifying parasitic infections and determining how well or how poorly your food is digested and obtaining other important information about your intestinal health.[3]

Although most physicians interested in yeast-related problems feel that laboratory tests do not "make the diagnosis of a candida-related health problem," other physicians I've consulted found that such studies may help. Two of my consultants, the late R. Scott Heath, a northern Kentucky/ Cincinnati neurologist and Dr. Robert Boxer, a Skokie, Illinois allergist, told me that the Candida Immune Complex test from AAL Reference Laboratory helped in evaluating and following their patients with yeast-related problems.[4]

You'll find a discussion of Dr. Heath's observations on pages 48–49 of the 2000 edition of *The Yeast Connection Handbook*. Other laboratories carrying out tests for *Candida albicans*, food allergies and nutritional deficiencies are listed in reference two and on pages 205–206 of *The Yeast Connection Handbook*.

REFERENCES

1. See the Candida Questionnaire and Score Sheet in Section VIII.

2. Burton Goldberg and the editors of *Alternative Medicine Guide to Chronic Fatigue, Fibromyalgia and Environmental Illness,* Future Medicine Publishers, Tiburon, CA, 1998, pp. 34–72.

3. You can obtain information about this test from Great Smokies Diagnostic Laboratory, 63 Zillicoa St., Asheville, NC 28801. 800-522-4762 or fax: 704-253-0621.

4. You can obtain additional information about the Candida Immune Complex test from AAL Reference Laboratory, 800-522-2611. Fax: 714-972-9979.

Water

Many articles in books today give you suggestions for overcoming your health problems. Most of them say, "You should drink 8 glasses of water each day." What kind of water should you drink and where should you get it? This question is pertinent because ordinary tap water may be contaminated with bacteria, parasites and other ingredients that can impair your health.

In a comprehensive cover story of the June 2000 issue of one of my favorite publications, *Nutrition Action Health Letter** David Schardt said,

> "The Environmental Protection Agency (EPA) requires water utilities to keep the levels of 80 potential contaminants below legal limits. But even when water meets all regulations it still may not be suitable for everyone to drink."

In his discussion Schardt reassured his readers when he said, "On the whole, Americans have good clean drinking water." Yet, he pointed out that while chlorinating water destroys many disease-causing bacteria, that chlorine, when combined with organic matter, forms compounds called disinfection byproducts (DBPs). And these DBPs may cause problems which are now being investigated.

Other problems with tap water cited by Schardt include turbidity, lead, arsenic and parasites. *When you read about them you'll*

---

*To obtain a copy of the 16-page issue of *Nutrition Action Health Letter* send your name, mailing information and $3 to CSPI, 1875 Connecticut Ave., N.W., Suite 300, Washington, DC 20009.

realize that you should not drink ordinary tap water without taking certain precautions. Here are some of Schardt's suggestions.

1. Use only water from the cold water tap for drinking and cooking. Hot water is likely to contain more lead and other metals. If the tap hasn't been turned on for six hours or more, run the water until it gets as cold as it's going to get. That helps flush out any metals that may have accumulated.

2. Purchase a pitcher or carafe that sits on your countertop or units that are mounted on your faucet. (Cost $10 to $75.) *It's important to remember that filters need to be replaced at a cost of $25 to $150 a year.*

3. You may also wish to investigate an under-the-sink unit which costs between $100 and $500. Here's how to choose a filter.

   ✦ Check to see if the filter has been tested and certified by NSF International, a nonprofit independent testing organization.
   ✦ Pick a standard. NSF's tests include Standard 42 which covers "aesthetic effects" which affect the water's taste, odor and color, but that are not considered harmful. Standard 53 covers "health effects" like reducing the parasite *Cryptosporidium,* lead, herbicides, pesticides, trihalomethanes—and many other contaminants "that may pose a health risk if present in water in concentrations that exceed allowable levels."

4. Check the contaminants. A filter is only certified to remove the contaminants that are listed on the box or in the package information.

How about spring water, mineral water, sparkling water and other bottled waters? You'll see bottles of these waters in every convenience store, gas station and supermarket. According to Schardt,

"Short of testing it yourself, there's no way to guarantee that bottle water is free of contaminants. But you improve your chances if you stick to brands bottled by companies that are members of the International Bottled Waters Association (IBWA). Their plants are open to unannounced inspection by NSF, an international independent certification agency."

You can obtain more information from IBWA by dialing their hotline (800-water11) or from their web page, www.bottled water.org. Other sources of information about water on the web are www.nsf.org and www.cspinet.org/nah/water.

More support for the importance of drinking water: In the August 2000 issue of _Health & Healing—Tomorrow's Medicine Today,_* the cover story article was entitled "Drink More Water!" Whitaker reviewed a number of reports in prestigious medical journals, as well as reports from his readers. All of them said that drinking more water improved the health of people with many disorders, including asthma, cancer, constipation, heart disease, stroke and kidney stones. In discussing the importance of water, Whitaker said,

"Think about it. Water makes up up to 70% of magnificently engineered bodies and while we can survive for months without food, we could last only days without water."

Whitaker referred to a book published several years ago by Fereydoon Batmanghelidj, M.D., _Your Body's Many Cries for Water._ Dr. Batmanghelidj proposed that dehydration is an underlying cause of most of the diseases afflicting mankind.

According to this physician, among the conditions increased water intake helps included neck and back pain. Here are some of Whitaker's "Recommendations for Water."

---

*For more information about this monthly publication, _Dr. Julian Whitaker's Health & Healing,_ call 800-539-8219.

- "Drink a minimum of 64 ounces of water every day. . . Don't wait until you're thirsty to drink—you'll likely never get this much down. Instead, keep filled water bottles at your desk, in your car, by your bed and by your favorite chair as a reminder.
- If you have congestive heart failure or kidney disease, or if you're taking diuretics, talk to your doctor before increasing your water intake."

SECTION

VI

COMMENTS BY OTHERS

Sidney M. Baker, M.D.

I met Sid Baker for the first time over 20 years ago. Since that time he's generously shared his knowledge and experiences with me on countless occasions. If you read my 1986 book *The Yeast Connection,* you may recall that I used a number of his concepts in Section C, "Keeping Candida Under Control Requires More Than Medication." I especially loved his discussion and drawing entitled "The Causes of Illness Resemble a Web" (Pages 39–46). You'll find many references to Dr. Baker's observations elsewhere of this book. (See Index for page numbers.)

In the introduction to his book *The Circadian Prescription,*[1] Baker said,

> "We're not only what we eat, but when we eat. . . At the core of my program is the Circadian diet, a powerful but simple eating plan that enables you to give your body the food it needs *when it needs it,* as dictated by the laws of circadian rhythm. Put simply, you will be eating most of your protein at breakfast and lunch and the bulk of your carbohydrates in the evening."

In answering the question "What is circadian rhythm?" Baker said it refers to your body's internal clock which completes a rhythmic cycle about every 24 hours. In his continuing discussion he said,

> "Not only do humans have circadian rhythms but also these rhythms are arranged sequentially. On a farm, the farmer wakes up, milks the cows, has breakfast, feeds the chickens and goes about his daily chores in a certain order; if he didn't the

animals would suffer and the farm wouldn't operate smoothly. Similarly, your body performs specific biochemical activities in a regular order that's repeated every day. You couldn't function if it didn't. . .

"Complaints such as fatigue, difficulty concentrating, depression, digestive and sleep disturbances, and other forms of mild malaise are . . . very common and troublesome for millions of people. *The Circadian Prescription* will help you tackle all of these problems."

In a further discussion of his "circadian prescription story" Baker told his readers to eat a varied diet rather than a limited number of foods. And he emphasizes fresh fruits and fresh vegetables because they provide fiber, antioxidants and plant pharmaceuticals which protect you against many diseases.

Among his interesting recommendations is the "rhythmic shake," which he says is the keystone of the diet. And he gives readers recipes for several different shakes, including his basic shake which contains 3 oz. of whole milk, 3 oz. of regular yogurt, 1 tablespoon of ground flax seeds, 3 tablespoons of soy protein isolate and one-fourth cup of fresh or frozen blueberries. The ingredients are blended at low speed initially and the speed is increased until the ingredients are "well blended."

For people who are sensitive to milk products he recommends shakes which contain soy milk or flax seed powder.

REFERENCE

1. Baker, S.M., *The Circadian Prescription*, Putnam, New York, 2000.

James H. Brodsky, M.D.

Dr. Brodsky,* a practicing internist, became interested in yeast-related disorders in the early 1980s and has been my friend and consultant since that time. In the Foreword to the 1986 paperback edition of *The Yeast Connection,* he said,

> "It is time for all physicians and medical scientists to increase their understanding of the relationship between yeast and human illness. Many patients with yeast-related health disorders are being treated ineffectively just because their problem has gone unrecognized. If one reviews the literature carefully, the supporting research is well documented."[1]

Brodsky reviews a dozen articles in the peer-reviewed literature which provided documentation, including reports by professionals in the U.S. and the U.K. In his concluding paragraph he said,

> "Enteric candida undoubtedly plays a greater role in human illness than has been previously suggested. A history of food and chemical intolerances is frequently seen in patients with a history of recurrent candida infections. There's increasing evidence that gut yeast may have a role in some instances of psoriasis.[2] Changes in mood and behavior related to yeast have been observed for over 30 years and reviewed by Iwata.[3]

---

*Brodsky is a Diplomate of the American Board of Internal Medicine; an instructor at Georgetown University Medical School; American College of Physicians; American Society of Internal Medicine.

Professionals must take note about what is known about the yeast/human interaction. We must help our patients overcome this illness which for most is probably iatrogenic* in origin."

In the Foreword to my book, *The Yeast Connection and the Woman,* Brodsky said,

"During the past decade, we've learned a great deal about chronic fatigue and the importance of listening to and not dismissing patients who complain of it. Many individuals with chronic fatigue immune dysfunction syndrome (CFIDS) have responded well to treatment for yeast, suggesting there may be a relationship between yeast and this illness. Cognitive impairment, sometimes described as spaciness, poor memory, or loss of concentration, is an all too common complaint. After other causes . . . have been systematically excluded, a trial of yeast-reduction therapy is suggested and is often remarkably effective."[4]

REFERENCES

1. Crook, W.G., *The Yeast Connection,* Professional Books, Jackson, Tennessee and Vintage Books, New York, NY, 1986.

2. Rosenberg, E. W., et al., "Response to Crohn's Disease in Psoriasis," *New England Journal of Medicine,* 308:101, 1983.

3. Iwata, K., "A review of the literature on drunken symptoms due to yeasts in the gastrointestinal tract," in Iwata, K. (ed.), "Yeast and Yeast-like Microorganisms in Medical Science," Tokyo, University of Tokyo Press, 1976, pp. 260–268.

4. Crook, W.G., *The Yeast Connection and the Woman,* Professional Books, Jackson, Tennessee, 1995/1998.

*Caused by physicians.

The CFIDS Chronicle

During the mid and late 1990s I've learned many things about chronic fatigue syndrome (CFS) from *The CFIDS Chronicle** published by The CFIDS Association of America, Inc. I also make annual donations to help this organization in its continuing work.

In the Reader's Forum section of the November/December 1998 issue of *The CFIDS Chronicle,* Janet Dauble, head of Share, Care and Prayer, Inc., P.O. Box 2080, Frazier, CA 93225, said,

> "Thank you, Dr. Cheney, for recommending elimination diets (July/August 1998, page 13). *In our experience with hundreds of people with disabling fatigue, cognitive problems and pain, finding out what foods they have become sensitive to and avoiding them has been the most helpful treatment tool of all.* And it is important to understand, as you pointed out, that a person can be very food allergic and not know it because of delayed and chronic reactions.
>
> "Of course, avoiding sugar, dairy and/or grains, etc. is not as easy as taking a pill, and it is not a quick cure. But a diet geared to each individual's sensitivities can often get him out of bed and give him his life back. It is also important to avoid using scented products, strong cleaning products and commercial pesticide/herbicides. Just using old fashioned cleaning products such as baking soda, vinegar, Bon-Ami and Borax can make a big difference for some persons with CFIDS (PWCs)."

Here are excerpts from the November/ December 1999 issue of *The CFIDS Chronicle.* In his message, Marc M. Iverson, MBA,

---

*The CFIDS Chronicle is published by The CFIDS Association of America, Inc., P.O. Box 220398, Charlotte, NC 28222–0398.

CPA, Chairman and Founder of The CFIDS Association of America, Inc., said,

> "It is crucial that we bring knowledge of promising emerging science to physicians as well as patients. To this end, we are planning for a medical newsletter on CFIDS, which will make its debut early next year. The newsletter will be mailed to health care professionals to enhance the legitimacy of CFIDS as a serious medical condition and keep them informed of progress on research and treatment. Association members also will receive the newsletter in addition to the *Chronicle* . . .
>
> "Another way the Association works to accelerate the pace of research is by advocating for it on Capitol Hill. We are fighting to ensure that CFIDS has a place on the national research agenda . . . Recently our efforts paid off when Congress directed the Centers for Disease Control and Prevention to return the entire $12.9 million that it misspent to the CFIDS research program. We continue to work to ensure that these restored funds—as well as any other CFIDS research funds—are used in ways that will help us solve the mysteries of this illness as soon as possible."

In this same issue of the *Chronicle,* Vicki C. Walker reviewed presentations of the Second World Congress on chronic fatigue syndrome (CFS) and related disorders, (Brussels, Belgium, September 9–12, 1999). In her review she discussed several of the 55 presentations and said that the proceedings will be published in the peer-reviewed *Journal of Chronic Fatigue Syndrome.* Here are excerpts from Walker's article.

> "The primary reason CFIDS patients have difficulty remembering things is because they have neurological impairments that hinder both learning and retrieving memories from storage, reported John Deluca, Ph.D. of Kessler Hospital in New Jersey.
>
> "In a recent study he conducted, 51 CFIDS patients required more time and study to commit facts to memory than

healthy individuals. Once they had memorized those facts, their ability to recall them was also impaired."

Walker also reviewed a discussion of Gulf War Illness (GWI) by Benjamin Natalson, M.D., Paul Levine, M.D., and Garth Nicolson, Ph.D. Dr. Natelson noted that GWI patients with Post-Traumatic Stress Disorder (PTSD) had a subnormal cardiovascular response to laboratory stressors. And he hypothesized that exposure to toxins or other pathogens during the War may have altered these veterans' stress responses.

Dr. Levine reported that the combination of four neurologic symptoms—blurred vision, balance/dizziness, tremor/shaking and speech difficulty were significantly more common in Gulf War veterans than in non-Gulf veterans.

Garth Nicolson discussed mycoplasma infections in GWI patients and found that 45% of GWI veterans and 65% of CFIDS and fibromyalgia patients have mycoplasma infections "which can be treated with antibiotics, although they're difficult to cure."

A further discussion of Dr. Nicolson's observations was published in the September/October 1999 issue of *The CFIDS Chronicle*.

In his 3-page article, "The Role of Microorganisms in Chronic Illness: Support for antibiotic regimens," Dr. Nicolson, Chief Scientific Officer and Research Professor at the Institute for Molecular Medicine in Huntington Beach, CA, said that this lab and the lab of others found that "about 60% of more than 200 civilians with CFIDS and FM showed infectious species of mycoplasma, especially *M. fermentans*."

He said that by contrast these infections are found in less than 10% of healthy controls. In discussing treatment with antibiotics, Nicholson said, "The recommended treatment for mycoplasmal blood infections requires long-term antibiotic therapy." He listed five different broad-spectrum antibiotics and said that multiple six-week cycles of treatment are usually necessary.

In his continuing discussion, he said,

"Some patients recover to a certain point and then fail to continue to respond to the recommended antibiotics, suggesting that other problems, such as viral infections, environmental exposure and other toxic events also may play an important role in these illnesses, and may even play a predominant role in some patients."

I've had no experience in treating patients with CFS/CFIDS using prolonged courses of antibiotic drugs. Yet, because antibiotics eradicate normal gut flora while they're wiping out enemies, they also promote the overgrowth of *Candida albicans* and abnormal bacteria, including *Clostridium difficile*.

Based on thousands of phone calls and letters I've received during the last 15 years, repeated courses of antibiotics, including long-term therapy (as for example antibiotics for acne, sinusitis, urinary or respiratory infections and Lyme Disease) play an important role in causing people to develop yeast-related disorders.

If for whatever reason a person is given broad-spectrum antibiotic drugs, I feel she/he should also receive probiotics, including *Lactobacillus acidophilus* and *Bifidobacterium bifidus* and the safe antifungal medication, nystatin. And in some individuals with yeast-related problems, Diflucan and/or other systemic antifungal drugs may be indicated. These agents, which discourage the overgrowth of *Candida albicans* in the gut, can be continued for a number of days, or even weeks after the antibiotic has been discontinued.

Search for a Test: In part one of the cover story article in the Winter 2000 issue of the *CFIDS Chronicle* entitled "The Search for the Test," Renée Brehio and Carol Sieverling said,

"Currently the diagnosis of chronic fatigue and immune dysfunction syndrome (CFIDS) involves eliminating all other possible causes, a lengthy process that is often expensive and painful. A proven diagnostic test would help erase doubts that CFIDS is real, as well as help physicians better identify the illness, begin treatment earlier and possibly shed some light on the cause.

"For years, researchers have been chasing this elusive Holy Grail. Most of the hunt has focused around trying to find a biochemical abnormality in CFIDS patients—something that can be found simply in urine or blood samples. On the surface, it seems that this should be a fairly easy task. It is obvious that many of the body systems of persons with CFIDS (neurological , immune and endocrine, just to name a few) do not function in a normal fashion. So why do we not have a test yet?

"One reason lies in the very existence of those multiple defects. Many different abnormalities have been found to be involved in CFIDS, so research needs to sort out the ones that could be tested for easily and reliably."

In their continued discussion, Brehio and Sieverling* described several tests that are now being studied including the enzyme RNase L which several researchers had found to be positive in the great majority of patients with CFIDS. Yet they said, "Despite this high accuracy, the researchers emphasize that the test cannot yet be considered a diagnostic marker. People with other illnesses may also have a high percentage of the defective enzyme."

They also discussed experimental tests for RNA which has been found in the sera of Gulf War veterans and 5-HIAA, a metabolite of serotonin, a neurotransmitter known to be responsible for mediating mood, sleep, perception and appetite.

I do not deny that tests of many types are important in studying people with fatigue, headache, depression, chemical sensitivities, abdominal pain and muscle aches. In my experience, these symptoms develop from multiple causes. I'd like to repeat

_____

*Renée Brehio is Director of Communications for the CFIDS Association of America. Carol Sieverling is Leader of the CFS/FM Support Group of Dallas/Ft. Worth.

the comments of my friend and mentor, Sidney M. Baker, M.D., who said in effect,

> "When a person is ill, we need to always ask ourselves these two questions: *Is there something this patient lacks that he/she needs? Is there some toxic, allergic or environmental substance that is making him/her sick?*"

Alexander Chester, M.D.

During a visit to Washington, D.C. in the early 1990s, I had lunch with this board-certified internist. I was delighted and excited to learn of his interest in food allergies/sensitivities and chronic fatigue syndrome. Since that time I've learned more about his interest in chronic sinusitis and its relationship to chronic fatigue. Here are excerpts from his letter published in the Spring 1995 issue of the *CFIDS Chronicle*.

"Most chronic fatigue is treated by internists who, as a group, have received little information about sinusitis in their training.[1] Large internal medicine and medical subspecialty texts often devote little more than a paragraph to chronic sinusitis. None mention it as a possible cause of chronic fatigue.

"Other sources of information, however, clearly indicate that chronic sinusitis can cause serious fatigue.[2] In *Sinus Survival*, the author states: 'There is scarcely a sinus patient I can think of who doesn't complain of some degree of fatigue. . . . At times, fatigue is the chief complaint.'[3] One of the earliest references linking sinusitis and fatigue was by Dr. Sam Roberts, Chief of Otolaryngology at the University of Kansas.[4]

"In a retrospective study of over 4000 patients he noted a very high prevalence of fatigue in those with sinus complaints. *Eighty-seven percent of the adult patients with chronic sinus problems noted some fatigue, with 'complete exhaustion' in 50 percent. It is hard to overstate the importance of making sure that a treatable disease is not overlooked in individuals devastated by fatigue.*[5] (emphasis added)

In discussing chronic sinusitis in a 1996 article published in *American Family Physician,* Dr. Chester said that chronic sinusitis is the most prevalent chronic condition in the United States and affects almost 32 million people. In discussing symptoms he said that those that are considered "classic" include facial pain, nasal congestion, discharge and cough—especially at night. He also said that people with sinusitis may feel a sensation of pressure in the face and in other areas of the head which is often worse in the morning. He said,

> "Additional complaints may include fatigue, dysequilibrium, dental pain, asthma, inability to focus mentally, minor visual changes and temporomandibular joint symptoms."[6]

In discussing therapy he said that the contribution of food allergies to chronic sinusitis is "controversial." In his extensive review of the medical literature he referred to a 1945 article by Theron Randolph who noted the coincidence of allergic disease, unexplained fatigue and enlarged lymph glands.[7]

In a 1999 report in *Medical Crossfire,* Chester and four other physicians participated in a debate on chronic fatigue syndrome. Here's an excerpt from the introduction to that article.

> "Characterized by the new onset of fatigue and flu-like symptoms, chronic fatigue syndrome (CFS) is a debilitating illness whose symptoms may persist or recur for years. Despite almost 15 years of substantial research efforts, the etiology of CFS remains obscure. Although CFS is now widely accepted as a valid diagnosis by most health care providers, there's still considerable disagreement as to its cause, diagnosis, and optimal management."

Participants other than Dr. Chester* in the discussion included Dr. David Bell, a Lyndonville, New York, family physi-

_____

*Dr. Alexander Chester, Clinical Professor of Medicine, Georgetown University Medical Center, Washington, D.C.

cian, Dr. Paul Levine, Clinical Professor of Medicine at George Washington University Medical Center, Dr. Peter Rowe, Professor of Pediatrics at Johns Hopkins School of Medicine (Baltimore) and Dr. Benjamin Natelson, Department of Neurosciences, University of Medicine and Dentistry of New Jersey (Newark). Here's another excerpt from the article.

> "Dr. Chester proposed chronic sinusitis as another important cause of severe fatigue. 'If you look at the number of criteria for chronic fatigue, many of them are compatible with a sinus or nasal cause: sore throats, tender cervical glands, headaches, dizziness and even fatigue.' He also referred to a study . . . that used a validated survey instrument and noted significant, serious fatigue and bodily pain . . . in those with sinusitis."[8]

My Comments: I was delighted to read about Dr. Chester's observations on sinusitis for a number of reasons, including his comments about the relationship of food allergies to this common problem. Many years ago (when I was a medical student at the University of Virginia) I took my meals at a boarding house where they put pitchers of cow's milk on the table. Instead of drinking water, I drank milk.

About that time I developed persistent nasal congestion and sinusitis. I went to Student Health and the physician in charge said, "Mr. Crook, your sinuses are blocked." A short time later, Dr. Fletcher Woodard, head of the ENT Department at UVa carried out a submucous resection (a type of nasal surgery). Although it was supposed to help, my sinuses continued to be congested.

Some years later, during my residency training in Baltimore, an otolaryngologist at Johns Hopkins put radium rods in my nose to lessen the congestion. (Ugh!) Then after I entered practice in Tennessee in the 1950s my problems with sinusitis continued until I visited Dr. Theron Randolph in 1955. During our visit, Dr. Randolph noted that I was rubbing my nose and clearing my throat. When he learned that cow's milk was my favorite beverage he said, "Dr. Crook, *I think that milk could be causing your nasal congestion and sinus problems.*" *I stopped drinking milk 45 years ago and my sinus symptoms were relieved. Since then they've only returned when I consumed too many dairy products.*

Another reason I became even more interested in Dr. Chester's observations: In a 1999 Mayo Clinic report otolaryngologist, Jens U. Ponikau, M.D., and colleagues, in a research study stated that the great majority (96%) of 200 consecutive patients with chronic rhinosinusitis showed positive fungal cultures[9]. Although *Candida albicans* wasn't among the fungi they identified, based on their observations and those of Dr. Chester, I feel that people with sinus complaints and chronic fatigue will benefit from a treatment program which includes a sugar-free special diet and Diflucan or other systemic oral antifungal medication.

I became even more interested in the sinus-fatigue connection in December 2000, just before sending this book to the printer. While browsing through Waldenbooks looking for Christmas presents for my daughters, I saw the revised and updated fourth edition of Dr. Robert Ivker's book *Sinus Survival*.* I was delighted to see that many pages of this book focused on *Candida albicans*. My Candida Questionnaire and Score Sheet (pages 218–222), Success Stories (pages 333–335, 338–341) and a discussion of "Extreme Fatigue" (pages 60–61) were included.

If you're bothered by sinus problems, even if you aren't

_____

*Robert S. Ivker, D.O., has been a family physician for thirty years. He is an assistant clinical professor in the Department of Family Medicine and a clinical instructor in the Department of Otolaryngology at the University Colorado School of Medicine, and past president of the American Holistic Medical Association.

"tired—so tired," read Dr. Ivker's book. According to the book cover, this book *"offers the most current holistic medical advice for the treatment, prevention and cure of sinusitis, allergies and colds."*

REFERENCES

1. Chester, A.C., "Chronic sinusitis and the internist: Inadequate training and education," *Arch. Intern. Med.*, 1994, 154:133–135.

2. Goldman, J.L., Blaugrund, S.M., Shugar, J.M., (eds.), *The Principles and Practice of Rhinology: A Text on the Diseases and Surgery of the Nose and Paranasal Sinuses,* John Wiley and Sons, New York, 1987.

3. Ivker, R.S., *Sinus Survival,* Putnam Publishing Group, New York, 1992, p. 28.

4. Roberts, S.E., "A new sinus syndrome," *Trans. Amer. Acad. Ophal. Otolaryngology,* 1945, 49:177–193.

5. Chester, A.C., "Chronic fatigue of nasal origin: Possible confusion with chronic fatigue syndrome." In: B. M. Hyde (ed.), *The Clinical and Scientific Basis of ME/CFS,* The Nightingale Research Foundation, Ottawa, 1992, pp. 260–266.

6. Chester, A.C., "Chronic Sinusitis," *American Family Physician,* Vol. 53, pp. 877–887, February 15, 1996.

7. Randolph, T.G., Hettig, R.A., "The coincidence of allergic disease, unexplained fatigue and lymphadenopathy; possible confusion with infectious mononucleosis," *Am. J. Med. Science,* 1945, 209:306–14.

8. Gliklich, R.E. and Metson, R., "The Health Impact of Chronic Sinusitis in Patients Seeking Otolaryngologic Care," *Otolaryngol. Head Neck Surg.*, 1995, 113:104–109.

9. Ponikau, J. U., et al., "The Diagnosis and Incidence of Allergic Fungal Sinusitis," Mayo Clinic Proc., 1999, 74:877–884.

Connecticut CFIDS
and FM Association

During the mid 1990s I was invited to make a presentation to members of this organization* at their conference in Hartford. Since that time I've been impressed by the information they present to readers in their newsletter. They held their annual spring conference in April 2000 at the University of Connecticut Health Center.

Miryam Ehrlich Williamson,† author of several books, including *Fibromyalgia—A Comprehensive Approach* and *The Fibromyalgia Relief Book* was the first speaker. In her talk Williamson told the audience her personal history which included her history of fibromyalgia which began at the age of five and developed to the point where she was bedridden in 1989. Here are excerpts from her presentation as reported by Michelle Lapuk, Co-president, Connecticut CFIDS and FM Association.

> "Because she is not a physician, she entitled her talk: 'Managing Fibromyalgia, A Nonmedical Approach—A Patient's Guide to Do-It-Yourself Health Care.' She discussed ways to improve the quality of one's life. Miryam does see a value in medical treatment, but she believes the patient must take control of their own health, calling her own approach do-it-

---

*The Connecticut CFIDS & FM Association is a charitable, not for profit association. To join this organization and receive their newsletter, send a $25 donation for a one-year membership to the Connecticut CFIDS & FM Association, Inc., P.O. Box 3010, Milford, CT 06460, 1-800-952-2037.

†Miryam can be reached for further questions at miryam@mwilliamson.com; or visit her web page www.mwilliamson.com. She takes calls between 4:00 and 6:00 P.M. at 798-544-7010.

yourself health care. Patients must learn everything they can about their condition. They must also make up their mind that they CAN feel better. . .

"She believes that CFIDS and FM have many similar symptoms, but may have different causes. . . When it comes to lifestyle changes, it does not really matter which you have as long as you see improvement in the quality of your life. She stressed the importance of building a support system and being your doctor's consultant. Although she recommended finding a support group, she said if you come home feeling dejected, look for other answers, including a buddy. She also suggested trying auxiliary medical personnel such as physical therapists and cognitive behavioral specialists. Patience and persistence are crucial, along with a divide and conquer attitude. . .

"There are many key factors to improvement. Many of them are common sense, but sometimes they're hard to implement. Improving diet and nutrition, pain management, sleep hygiene, moderate exercise, body work, such as message, and attitude and stress management. . . Be aware of food allergies and sensitivities. Try an elimination diet to see if you feel better. Also, drink plenty of water. When you're thirsty you already may be dehydrated. Drink, drink, drink.

"If you have food cravings, especially for carbohydrates, you may be allergic to them. Try elimination in this area as well and see if symptoms improve. Many fibromyalgia patients have problems with malabsorption. Miryam feels this malabsorption may be caused by yeast overgrowth. . .

"When the complexity of FM gets you down, you need to divide and conquer. Pick one problem, work and focus on it. Try to improve in stages. List your options and try one thing and then another. You must have a game plan. Keep records and chart your progress. . . Don't give up. You're the expert on your body. You know what is best for you. Don't waste energy defending yourself or convincing others. Try to stay focused on your goal and ways to achieve it."

Elmer M. Cranton, M.D.

first met Dr. Cranton in 1971 at a health conference in Florida. Subsequently, we became members of the Advisory Board of Nathan Pritikin's Longevity Research Institute in California. I visited him on several occasions in the 1980s and 1990s and have sought his advice and consultation countless times. I've referred to his observations in all of my books. Here are his comments about yeast-related illness which I adapted from his discussion on the Internet.

"Multiple symptoms of a seemingly unrelated nature, often misdiagnosed as neurotic, are caused by immune system dysfunction related in part to an increase in body levels of *Candida albicans* and other fungal organisms. Treatments which reduce levels of yeasts and other fungi in the body and, thus, remove stress from the immune system, will bring improvement to a large majority of patients who have been unresponsive to multiple treatment programs elsewhere. This type of illness is increasingly prevalent and often unrecognized by the medical profession.

"Descriptive diagnostic terms variously used include Chronic Fatigue and Immune Dysfunction Syndrome (CFIDS), chronic fatigue syndrome, chronic Epstein-Barr virus syndrome, myalgic encephalomyelitis (ME), environmental illness, hypoglycemia, premenstrual syndrome, food and chemical sensitivity and food allergy. Most such terms imply immune dysfunction and in some cases hormonal imbalance.

"The most common and incapacitating symptom is profound and prolonged fatigue, without another plausible cause. Depression is commonly present, and often severe. Physical examination and laboratory tests seldom point to a definite diagnosis. Incorrect diagnoses often include psychoneurosis, hypochondriasis and endogenous depression. Adverse reactions to many nutritious foods (so-called food allergy) is common, as well as unusual sensitivity to chemical fumes, and respiratory allergy of the hay fever type. Stomach, intestinal, urinary, reproductive, muscle and joint symptoms are common.

"When seeking treatment, it's important to find physicians and nurses who understand CFIDS and provide a compassionate setting for treatment. Effective treatment consists of multiple antifungal medications prescribed together, avoidance of the most reactive foods and environmental exposures, an antifungal diet and supplemental vitamins, minerals and trace elements. In Dr. Cranton's experience, this program relieves stress and provides nutritional support for the impaired immune system."*

*Adapted from Cranton, E., Yeast-Related Illness & Chronic Fatigue and Immune Dysfunction Syndrome, www.drcranton.com.

Mary Enig, Ph.D.

n a paragraph in the introduction to her book, *Know Your Fats: The Complete Primer for Understanding the Nutrition of Fats, Oils and Cholesterol,* Dr. Enig* said,

"As we close the second millennium, the prevailing clinical approach from both the nutrition and medical communities in the United States has condemned a high dietary intake of almost all fats. This emphasis on reducing dietary fat intake has developed from concerns about diet serum cholesterol/coronary heart disease (CHD) and dietary fat/cancer relationships that have emanated from organizations such as the American Heart Association . . . and the U.S. Department of Agriculture's Dietary Guidelines (and many others)."

In her discussion she said that some recent research reports show that saturated fatty acids found in natural food could be good for you and that low fat diets cause health problems of many types. She especially targeted the partially hydrogenated fats and oils which are high in *trans* fatty acids. "These fatty acids are mostly the unnatural kind that accumulate in our bodies and cause disease."

In discussing cholesterol, she said that it "is perhaps the most misunderstood and wrongly maligned biological molecule in existence." She points out our brains are largely cholesterol and saturated fats and that infants who don't get enough cholesterol

---

*Dr. Mary Enig received her M.S. and Ph.D. in Nutritional Sciences from the University of Maryland. She has served as president of the Maryland Nutritionists Association; and is a Fellow of the American College of Nutrition. Dr. Enig's book is published by Bethesda Press, Silver Spring, Maryland. Fax: 301-680-8100. www.bethesdapress.com.

during their first years when their brains are developing, risk a loss of cognitive function. The bottom-line message from her discussion: *Fear of cholesterol is unwise.*

In discussing weight gain and/or loss, she said that the U.S. has more of an obesity problem than any other country, including people in countries where they consume only natural fats. In discussing dietary fat in children she asked, "What would you think of a total diet that supplied 53.5% of the calories of fat, of which 25.8% of the calories are saturated fat?" She said this is the typical diet of the breast-fed infant from a well-nourished mother. She asked and answered the question, "Are we eating too much fat?" She said that humans, including growing children, need *substantial* amounts of fats in their diet.

In answering the question "What are you to believe?" Dr. Enig said,

> "Unfortunately, a current driving philosophy among the food and nutrition scientists is that the food industry can improve on the natural foods. . . What seems so ironic is that the very foods (saturated fats and cholesterol) that people are avoiding, are the very foods that are helpful and health-giving. . . The healthy and smart bottom line—use a mixture of natural fats in moderation."

She recommends butter rather than margarine. *She says that canola oil and soybean oil (which are usually partially hydrogenated) should not be used.* Instead of these oils, for sautéing and light frying she uses a blend containing one-third olive oil, one-third sesame oil and one-third coconut oil. She said, "It is easy to make up in small portions ranging from a single tablespoon (1 tsp of each) to a pint and a half (1 cup of each)."

Leo Galland, M.D.

I met Leo Galland, a friend and former associate of Sid Baker, over 15 years ago. I've "picked his brain" on many occasions and cited and quoted his observations in all of my books.

In his book *Power Healing,* Dr. Galland discussed why people became ill and emphasized the importance of *precipitating events* and *triggers* which play an important role in causing a person to develop an illness. The triggers cited by Dr. Galland include trauma, exercise, microbes, drugs, toxins, allergens, foods, thoughts, images, memories, repetitive activities and social interactions.

> "*Triggers* are often not disease specific, however; they tend to be specific to the individual. Many chronic ailments have multiple interacting triggers."

One of Dr. Galland's patients had been ill for 18 months with fatigue, headaches, blurred vision and inability to exercise. Three years prior to his visit with Dr. Galland this patient had been strong and healthy. Then he became ill with pneumonia and was treated with multiple antibiotic drugs. Following this illness he developed digestive problems which hung on. In discussing this patient Dr. Galland said,

> "The precipitating event was clearly an acute illness, pneumonia. I suspected that the culprit was not the infection itself, but an effect of the antibiotic he had taken. One of the patterns that my colleagues and I repeatedly encountered during our investigation at the Gesell Institute was the development of chronic illness following the use of antibiotics. We thought that antibiotics might precipitate chronic disease by altering

the body's ecology. Each person is colonized by over 100 trillion bacteria . . . Destruction of these bacteria by antibiotics may be injurious, allowing the overgrowth of unfriendly organisms which proliferate when they are controlled by the normal flora."

When this patient was treated with a special diet, nystatin and a preparation of *Lactobacillus acidophilus,* after a period of several weeks his symptoms all disappeared and he has remained well for the past five years.

"The notion that yeast colonizing in the intestinal tract can cause symptoms such as fatigue or headache has generated heated controversy within the medical profession over the past few years . . . Opponents of the yeast theory have discussed the problem as if yeast overgrowth was supposed to be a new disease. It's nothing of the kind. It is a toxic reaction of a type that can occur with any infection, aggravated by the ability of yeast to generate strong allergic reactions in people they infect."[1]

REFERENCE

1. Galland, L., *Power Healing,* Random House, 1998, pp. 66–71.

Burton Goldberg

n a two-page article published in the *Washington Post* (Friday, January 28, 1994), Margaret Mason featured the 1068-page-book, *Alternative Medicine: The Definitive Guide.* According to Mason, this book was put together by Burton Goldberg, a 67-year-old developer who spent almost $2 million completing it. I received a copy of this book in early 1994 and later that year I met Goldberg at a health food convention in Baltimore. *I was truly impressed by his dedication and his desire to help people.*

Since that time, Goldberg and the editors of *Alternative Medicine* magazine have published a number of other books, including a 1998 book, *Alternative Medicine Guide to Chronic Fatigue, Fibromyalgia & Environmental Illness.*

This book includes a comprehensive discussion of alternative therapies which help people with chronic fatigue (CF), fibromyalgia (FM) and environmental illness (EI). Here are excerpts from the introduction to this book entitled "You Don't Have to Endure **Chronic Fatigue**."

"If you have CHRONIC FATIGUE syndrome or one of its close relatives—fibromyalgia and environmental illness—you most likely have experienced years of frustration trying to find relief from your puzzling assortment of symptoms. You may have spent years just trying to find a doctor who could tell you what's wrong with you. In the process, you've probably encountered many medical professionals who dismiss your complaints as 'neurotic imaginings. . . .'

". . .the whole conventional medical establishment . . . has spent the past decade squabbling over whether CFS even exists and, if it does, debating the number and nature of symptoms that qualify a person for the distinction of having CFS. This has been the pursuit of the U.S. government's Center for Disease Control whose accomplishments after more than ten years of investigating CFS consist of the development of formal diagnosis criteria.

"But they are no closer to discovering what causes CFS (or how to treat it) than they were when the outbreak in Incline Village, Nevada, first drew their attention in the mid-1980s to what would become an epidemic. Conventional medical research, as it does with most illnesses, seems capable only of focusing on the search for that single cause which will then yield the mythical magic bullet cure. That's not the way alternative medicine goes about dealing with a complex illness like chronic fatigue.

"The good news is that you don't have to wait for the magic bullet because it will never arrive. Alternative medicine has practical solutions for you _now_. The reason is that physicians of alternative medicine know that illness is _multifactorial_. Especially in the case of such complex disorders as CFS, fibromyalgia and environmental illness, no one cause is responsible. Multiple imbalances and deficiencies combine to produce the breakdown of the body."

In this book you'll find a discussion of many different therapies, including the comments of 26 doctors who tell how they treat their patients. Among the many topics discussed are:

hidden thyroid problems	allergies
heavy metal toxicity	nutritional deficiency
parasites	candidiasis

You can find this book and other of Goldberg's books in health food stores and some bookstores, or you can obtain it by calling 800-333-4325. Goldberg also maintains a comprehensive website at www.alternativemedicine.com.

Anthony L. Komaroff, M.D.

I n the Spring 2000 issue of *The CFS Research Review,* in an article entitled "The Physical Basis of CFS," Dr. Komaroff said,

"Often when people hear that there is no known test or cause for chronic fatigue syndrome (CFS), they mistakenly understand that to mean that the illness isn't real. This is incorrect.

"Over the past 15 years scientists have identified numerous biological abnormalities that provide evidence for the reality and seriousness of CFS, even though the cause of CFS and diagnostic tests for it are still unknown.

"These biological abnormalities have given researchers clues to the cause of the illness. In particular, they have provided evidence that the illness involved both the brain and the immune system.

"There are no diagnostic tests yet for CFS because none of the biological abnormalities clearly distinguishes patients with CFS from other individuals. In reality, there are no perfect biological tests for any illness.

"When a test gets close enough to perfect, clinicians use it to help confirm or refute their clinical judgment. Testing in CFS has primarily been used to rule out other illnesses that can also cause chronic fatigue."

In his continuing discussion, Dr. Komaroff discussed the possible causes of CFS, including the cases which begin with "symptoms suggesting an infection, like a common viral illness." He cited several research reports which indicate that "no single infectious agent is likely to be *the* cause of CFS. Instead, CFS is likely to be caused by some abnormality in the body's response to any of several different infectious agents."

He also pointed out that "some infectious agents permanently live in a dormant state inside our bodies" and appear to "get reawakened in patients with CFS." He also reviewed various immune system abnormalities and neurological findings which are found in patients with CFS and he pointed out that epidemiological data "has helped to establish the relevance and importance of CFS as a serious public health issue."

In his concluding paragraph entitled **"CFS Is Real,"** Dr. Komaroff said that there are now scientific observations which "provide important evidence that CFS is not 'all in the head' or an imagined illness."

George F. Kroker, M.D.

This board-certified practicing physician has been my friend and consultant for over 20 years. I've sought his help and consultation on numerous occasions. He and his wife, Leslie, wrote the Foreword to *The Yeast Connection Cookbook* and he wrote the Foreword to *The Yeast Connection Handbook*. Dr. Kroker is also a strong supporter of the International Health Foundation (IHF) and a member of the IHF Advisory Board.

In my 1995/1998 book, *The Yeast Connection and the Woman*, I included the following comments by Dr. Kroker.

"I'm writing in response to your request for my impressions in treating Candida Related Complex. As you know, I'm a university-trained board-certified physician. I treated my first patient with this illness in late 1978 after I missed the diagnosis in one of my patients and learned more about it from Dr. Orian Truss in Birmingham, Alabama.

"I became so intrigued as to why this illness had such diverse manifestations; as you know, I subsequently reviewed the classical literature on candida-related pathology and contributed a chapter on this subject to an allergy textbook. . ."[1]

"I've treated several thousand patients with this illness . . . [and] I've arrived at the following clinical impressions.

1. *Candida-related complex cannot be treated successfully without simultaneous attention to a sugar and yeast free diet.* (emphasis added)
2. *Candida-related complex often is associated with other illnesses, most notably mold allergy, chemical sensitivities, autoimmune*

thyroiditis, and food intolerances. Unless these illnesses are screened for, the treatment of Candida (antifungal medication and diet) may completely fail to ameliorate the patients' symptoms. I cannot overemphasize the importance of the 'total load' in dealing with these patients. This makes it hard to set up a study. (emphasis added)

3. *Candida-related complex* seems to be a chronic and relapsing illness in many patients. Patients have a remission in illness and need no antifungal medication and be more lenient on their diet, only to relapse and have a return to illness with stress, dietary indulgence, antibiotics, ...

   "Candida-related complex seems to co-exist frequently in patients with premenstrual syndrome and also in patients with chronic fatigue syndrome. Treating the candida illness seems to often improve both of these other problems.

4. *Unfortunately candida remains a disease in search of a laboratory test for diagnosis. The best test remains a history and a one-month trial of antifungal medication and diet. I've tried to utilize antibody assays, cultures, etc., and they all fall short of diagnostic certainty."*[2]

In my opinion, Dr. Kroker's comments are so comprehensive, yet so succinct that they "say it all." *I sincerely hope they will be carefully read and digested, not only by skeptical physicians, but also by people who feel their health problems are yeast related.*

REFERENCES

1. Kroker, G.F., "Chronic Candidiasis and Allergy," in Brostoff, J. and Challacombe, C., *Food Allergy and Intolerance,* Balliére Tindall, Eastbourne, England and W. B. Saunders, Philadelphia, PA, 1987, pp. 850–870.

2. Crook, W.G., *The Yeast Connection and the Woman,* Professional Books, Jackson, TN, 1995/1998, pp. 653–654.

Zoltan P. Rona, M.D., M.Sc.

first met this knowledgeable physician during a trip to Toronto in the 1980s. Since that time I've visited with him in person and on the phone on many occasions. Here are excerpts from his comprehensive and authoritative book, *Return to the Joy of Health*.

> "If you've been told you have CFS, the good news is there's a lot you can do to help yourself to a speedy recovery . . . Do not listen to negative people, medical or otherwise, who claim that nothing can be done or that you need to see a psychiatrist . . . While there's no specific, recognized medical treatment for CFS, one can dramatically improve the function of the immune system through good nutrition, antioxidant supplementation and supportive herbal or homeopathic remedies."

In his continuing discussion, Rona pointed out that the immune system requires healthier levels of many nutrients, including zinc, calcium, magnesium, selenium, B complex vitamins, especially B^5, B^6 and B^{12}. He also said that removing sugar and white flour products from the diet is often helpful with most of the signs and symptoms of CFS. In discussing the controversies and myths surrounding sugar, Rona said,

> "The only people saying that sugar is harmless are those involved in the sugar industry . . . The sugar controversy has nothing to do with science; it's strictly a political debate similar to the one involving the association between cigarette smoking and lung cancer raised in the 1950s and 1960s. It may take

another decade before the powerful sugar lobby takes the same battering that is presently being taken by the tobacco industry.

"Study after study demonstrates that sugar consumption is directly or indirectly associated with poor health. *The volume of supporting literature is staggering* . . . Sugar goes by many names, including sucrose, fructose, brown sugar, invert sugar, dextrose, maltose, lactose . . . honey and molasses. . . . Sugar is hidden in many commercially available foods. For example, 1 tablespoon of ketchup contains one teaspoon of sugar. Some soft drinks contain up to 12 teaspoons of sugar per eight fluid ounces. . . Mayonnaise, cereals, breads, mustard, relish, peanut butter, gravy, sausage, TV dinners, and even drugs, are hidden sources of large amounts of sugar."

As you might guess, I was pleased that Rona, in his own practice, found that many chronically ill people, including those who are tired, so tired, are helped by a comprehensive treatment program that includes antifungal medication.

He also said,

"There is little, if any, evidence to suggest that anyone suffering from candida syndrome must eliminate yeast from their diet in order to clear up symptoms . . . Admittedly there are rare individuals with strong sensitivity to yeast-containing foods, molds and fungi . . . Dr. William Crook agrees that most sufferers of candidiasis can keep yeast-containing foods and supplements in their diet."[1]

REFERENCE

1.   Zona, Z. P., *Return to the Joy of Health,* Alive Books, 1997, pp. 36–37, 47–49.

Bruce Semon,
M.D., Ph.D.

everal years ago I learned of the interest of this Wisconsin nutritionist and child psychiatrist in yeast-related problems. His interest had been stimulated mainly because he and his wife, Lori Kornblum, are parents of an autistic child who'd been helped by a treatment program which featured dietary changes and nystatin.* At the June 2000 meeting of the Wisconsin Chronic Fatigue Association, Dr. Semon discussed the relationship of yeast to chronic fatigue. Here's information which I excerpted and adapted from a handout he presented to those attending the conference.

"I have helped many sufferers of chronic fatigue syndrome by treating the yeast *Candida albicans*. Let me explain why this therapy helps. *Candida albicans* normally lives in the intestinal tract. It can also be found at times in the mouth and causes an infection commonly called thrush.

"Bacteria also live inside the intestinal tract, sharing space with the yeast. After a person takes antibiotics, yeasts grow to fill in the space left by the removal of bacteria. Even after the antibiotics have been stopped, yeasts continue to multiply. Pregnancy and birth control pills also promote the grow of yeast at a higher level.

"Yeasts make a number of chemical compounds which are then picked up and absorbed by the body. These toxic compounds adversely affect the nervous system and include toxic

---

*Because of Dr. Semon's success in helping his child and his patients, he and Lori Kornblum published a cookbook entitled, *Feast Without Yeast—4 Stages to Better Health*. For more information about this book call 877-332-7899.

alcohols, aldehydes and the nervous system poison hydrogen sulfide. Alcohols depress the nervous system and at least some aldehydes are anesthetic agents, which put the brain to sleep. These chemicals slow the brain down so that it no longer works correctly.

"Chemicals in the diet also cause adverse effects on the brain. Foods containing these chemicals include barley malt, the raw material for making beer. Vinegar also contains chemicals which play a part in causing fatigue. Literally these chemicals keep the body and brain from functioning at the normal level of energy. When these chemicals are removed, by changing the diet and treating the intestinal yeast, the body's energy returns.

"One way to reverse an intestinal yeast problem is to take the anti-yeast drug nystatin. . . Fortunately because nystatin is not absorbed it causes no harmful effects, except occasional nausea. . . *All the tired patients who changed their diets and took nystatin regained at least a part of their energy. Some of these people had been so fatigued they couldn't get out of bed. Even these patients improved.*" (emphasis added)

Stephen Sinatra, M.D.

In the July 2000 issue of his newsletter *Heart Sense,** Stephen Sinatra, M.D.[†], wrote a three-page discussion entitled "Help for Energy Loss and Chronic Fatigue Syndrome." Here are excerpts from his article.

"After heart disease one of the most common problems people tell me about in my clinic is a lack of energy. You'd be amazed at the scope of this trend. Increasingly younger and healthier people are affected. And, occasionally, I'll see someone with a full blown case of energy deprivation in the form of Chronic Fatigue Syndrome (CFS). . . Although we still don't know what causes CFS we're learning more about how to treat it. . . We also know that many of these treatments have application for people who suffer from less acute forms of energy loss."

In his discussion Sinatra reviewed many therapies which he's found useful in treating his patients, including essential fatty acids, CoQ_{10} and magnesium. He also talked about the role toxic chemicals may contribute to chronic fatigue and he said,

"Another way to reduce toxic chemicals in your body is to omit foods that come in cans or boxes. Most, if not all, of these processed foods are laced with chemicals that drain your

---

*Heart Sense is published monthly by Phillips Publishing, Inc., 7811 Montrose Rd., Potomac, MD 20854-3394. 800-211-7643.

†Sinatra is an Assistant Clinical Professor at the University of Connecticut School of medicine, a board-certified cardiologist and author of the newsletter *Heart Sense,* and a number of books, including *The Co-Q_{10} Phenomenon.* In his practice he integrates conventional medical treatments with complementary, nutritional and psychological therapies. For more information call his hotline, 301-738-8234.

immune system. To feel your best and fight CFS, plan a diet rich in fresh organic fruits and vegetables, lean range meats, and organic eggs. Consider juicing as well. Add soy and flax to your diet to get vital omega-3 essential fatty acids, and you've got a great dietary combination to combat CFS.

"Lastly, probiotics and prebiotics are key for good intestinal health. It's mind boggling to think that 80 percent of illnesses originate from toxins in the bowel."

Sinatra also focused on other therapeutic agents which he has found effective, including NADH. In his discussion he said that it makes sense to make a "frontal assault on CFS by increasing adenosine triphosphate (ATP), the 'energy of life.'" And without this substance, the energy systems would crumble within eight seconds. He said that NADH was one of the best biochemical supports for enhancing ATP production. In discussing this substance he said,

> "NADH . . . is a cofactor that mediates electron transport in the mitochondria. In other words, these tiny organelles are the powerhouses of cells that generate energy. NADH can be taken in a supplement, called Enada, that is sold in health food stores. . . Studies performed at Georgetown Medical Center demonstrated that patients taking 10 mg of Enada for only four weeks acknowledged a 31 percent symptom reduction and improved by 81 percent in one year. No side effects were noted."

He also recommended L-carnitine, which he said helps support mitochondria. In discussing this substance he said,

> "CoQ_{10} is the spark that ignites the ATP process and L-carnitine is the freight train that shuttles fatty acids to be burned as fuel into the mitochondria. Then, after the fatty acids are burned, L-carnitine removes the toxic metabolites (waste products) from the mitochondria, which keeps the cells at peak energy utilization."

Sinatra said the best biochemical support for enhancing ATP production includes CoQ_{10}, NADH, magnesium and L-carnitine—together a perfect recipe for fighting chronic fatigue syndrome.

Jacob Teitelbaum, M.D.

I n the mid-1990s, during a trip to Washington, D.C., this board certified internist and I had a one and a half hour visit. I was fascinated by some of the things he told me. During our conversation he said in effect,

> "When I was in medical school in the 1970s, following a nasty viral illness, I didn't feel well. And by the end of the month I was finding it impossible to get out of bed, even by noon. My own illness, including fatigue, aching, poor sleep and bowel problems, prompted me to make a lot of changes in my own life. And with my family and friends' help and support, and my own work, I recovered my energy and strength and went on to finish medical school and residency.
>
> "Although I did well for a while I continued to suffer from fatigue, achiness and poor sleep. So I began to study this illness which was affecting so many people."

Working with a colleague, Barbara Bird (his lab manager and research partner), Dr. Teitelbaum completed a placebo-controlled study of 70 patients with fibromyalgia/chronic fatigue syndrome using multiple therapies, including the antifungal drug, Sporanox. Patients in the treated group enjoyed "significantly greater benefit" when compared to the placebo group. (P = .0001.)

Because of his own personal experiences and the success he had in treating many patients with severe chronic fatigue and other disorders, in 1996 Dr. Teitelbaum published a classic book, *From Fatigued to Fantastic*. In this book, which is written for both patients and physicians, he described his program for managing CFS and fibromyalgia.

He especially emphasizes the importance of multiple therapies, all given simultaneously. These include treatment for yeast infections, hormone dysfunction, immune dysfunction, parasites and nutritional inadequacies.

In November 1999 I interviewed Dr. Teitelbaum. Here are brief excerpts from a typescript of our conversation.

Dr. C: What one or two therapeutic interventions do you feel are most important?
Dr. T: They're all important, but if I had to pick two I would begin with 7–8 hours of solid sleep a night without waking and treating the yeast. Although there are two main therapeutic interventions, there are over 20 different things that need to be treated.

Dr. C: In what percentage of your patients was the onset gradual and what percent sudden?
Dr. T: About 60% sudden; 40% gradual. In those with a sudden onset it's usually kind of a viral infection, like the flu that comes and never leaves. There are other infections that can trigger it as well. But again what happens with a lot of these patients is that when they're not better two weeks later they get course after course of antibiotics. It's also possible that some of these people have received a lot of antibiotics before they developed the viral infection. Such antibiotics set them up for yeast overgrowth and other problems. Then when they get the viral infection and more antibiotics, it pushes them over the edge.

Dr. C: How important are food allergies and the leaky gut?
Dr. T: I find that once I treat the yeast, parasites and adrenal hormone deficiency, most peoples' food allergies go away. The one place we differ in our treatment protocols is that I don't really need to use the yeast-free diet for most of my patients.

334

If I keep sugar out of the diet and treat the other problems, my patients improve.

Dr. C: You've obviously made a 100% recovery from your own problems.
Dr. T: MY own CFS has been a good teacher. It's not the enemy. It has taught me how to take care of myself properly.

Dr. C: Have you been harassed by the medical establishment because of your interest in yeast?
Dr. T: No. In fact, I've been asked to serve as a peer-reviewer for the Maryland State Medical Society.

You can learn more about Dr. Teitelbaum's experiences and treatment program from his book, _From Fatigued to Fantastic_. You can also pull up his web page at www.endfatigue.com.

C. Orian Truss, M.D.

This Alabama physician deserves the credit for first noting that seemingly benign *Candida albicans* infections were related to illnesses in many parts of the body. He published four articles describing this relationship in the 1970s and early 1980s, and a book, *The Missing Diagnosis*.

In a scientific report published in 1992, Dr. Truss and his colleagues carefully reviewed their experiences in treating 40 premenopausal women with chronic yeast vaginitis and a variety of generalized symptoms.

In their carefully conducted scientific studies, they compared the responses of patients treated with nystatin, diet and immunotherapy to those treated with a placebo. Here are excerpts from the abstract of their study.*

> *"Full treatment . . . led to highly significant . . . improvement in 24 of 25 general symptoms. . . Toxic, immunologic enzymatic and allergic mechanisms are suggested. A therapeutic trial of nystatin and diet will establish a diagnosis in six weeks or less."*[1]

In their discussion, "Yeast and the Chronic Fatigue Syndrome," they said,

> "The 'chronic fatigue syndrome' was defined in 1988 in a report issued jointly by a number of major medical institutions.[2] The symptoms reported closely parallel those described earlier in the superficial candidiasis syndrome[3]—symptoms relieved by nystatin, diet and immunotherapy.

---

*Address reprint requests to C. Orian Truss, M.D., Critical Illness Research Foundation, 2614 Highland Ave., Birmingham, AL 35205-1799.

"Additional indication for an etiological role for yeast in this symptoms-complex was the reported clearing of these symptoms with ketoconazole therapy and 84% of 1100 patients selected by the criteria set forth in the initial 'chronic fatigue syndrome' paper. Lending objectivity to these results (not blinded) was the fact that 685 of the 1100 patients were on disability prior to treatment with only 12 remaining on disability after several months of ketoconazole therapy. . .

"It was concluded that *C. albicans* was the cause of these symptoms 'in a great majority of cases.' The added therapeutic benefit of a low-carbohydrate diet was stressed. *One important result of the defining of this syndrome was to give legitimacy to these multiple complaints by patients who heretofore had so often been dismissed as psychoneurotic.*"[4] (emphasis added)

Here are excerpts from their conclusions.

"Chronic superficial yeast infections may lead to generalized symptoms. A 6-week therapeutic trial of nystatin and diet is adequate to establish or reject the diagnosis . . . This simple, safe and relatively inexpensive six-week therapeutic trial will identify yeast as the cause of this complex of symptoms and stop the very large expense entailed in the repeated investigation of these symptoms.

"Symptoms used to define 'the chronic fatigue syndrome' closely parallel those reported in association with chronic superficial yeast infections, and have been found to be relieved by the antiyeast drug nystatin and ketoconazole, each administered together with a low carbohydrate-low yeast diet."

REFERENCES

1. Truss, C.O., Truss, C.V. and Cutler, R.B., "Generalized Symptoms in Women with Chronic Yeast Vaginitis: Treatment with nystatin, diet and immunotherapy vs. nystatin alone," *Journal of Advancement in Medicine,* 5:139–175, 1992.

2. Holmes, G.P. et al., "Chronic Fatigue Syndrome: A working definition," *Ann. Int. Med.*, 1988; 108:387–389.

3. Truss, C.O., "Tissue Injury Induced by Candida albicans: Mental and neurologic manifestations," *J. Ortho. Psychiatry,* 1978; 7:17–37.

4. Jessop, C., Chronic Fatigue Syndrome Conference, *Chronic Fatigue Syndrome Quarterly,* April 15, 1989, San Francisco, CA and personal communication: July 16, 1989.

Andrew Weil, M.D.

Good Fats, Bad Fats was the feature story in the December 1998 issue of Dr. Weil's newsletter, *Self Healing*.* Here's a summary of some of the advice he gave to his readers.

+ Keep fat intake *moderately* low. (Between 25 and 30% of calories.)
+ Eat: (a) oily fish (preferably Alaskan wild salmon) canned sardines or herring, or fresh mackerel in season, several times a week.
  (b) one to two tablespoons of ground flax seeds every day.
  (c) a half cup of toasted hemp seeds.
  (d) a handful of plain or dry roasted walnuts.
+ Make olive oil your cooking oil of choice.
+ Rather than putting butter or margarine on your bread, try nonhydrogenated spreads made with olive or expeller pressed canola oil.
+ Feel free to snack on nuts occasionally.
+ Minimize your intake of bad fats whenever possible. These include saturated fats and polyunsaturated fats. Avoid trans fatty acids found in margarine, vegetable shortening, hydrogenated vegetable oils and products made from them
+ Avoid any product if the ingredients include partially hydrogenated oil. (Including virtually all commercial snack foods such as crackers, cakes, cookies, pastries and deep-fried foods).

*For more information about *Self Healing* call 1-800-523-3296.

Ray C. Wunderlich, Jr., M.D.

I n my 1986 book, *The Yeast Connection,* in a two-page statement entitled "A Special Message for the Physician," I included the comments of this Florida physician who said,

> "Desirable at all times, is a balanced approach that holds a healthy respect of *Candida albicans.* . . At the same time, one does not wish to overlook the many other health departures that invite the candida syndrome. Those who suspect that they have symptoms due to candida overgrowth must not plunge headlong into a quest for a 'magic bullet.' Best and most long lasting health will be fostered by a careful inquiry into yeast, but also, into psychological, nutritional, allergic, degenerative and toxic factors."[1]

During the past 14 years, Wunderlich and I have discussed our interests and observations in person, by mail and on the phone. I've been pleased because for several decades he's written about food allergies and the adverse effects of consuming sugar. He's also shared with me his own observations in managing his patients.

In 1997, he published a superb 48-page booklet, *The Candida-Yeast Syndrome—The spreading epidemic of yeast-connected diseases: how to recognize and deal with them.* Here are excerpts from his introduction.

> "The yeast connection now occupies center stage in the practices of nutritionally oriented doctors, nutritionists and many other therapists who see clearly the broad range of

factors that account for so much of the misery that their clients experience. For better or worse, health food store personnel have become resident experts on the condition because of the flock of individuals who patronize their stores seeking relief when their doctors fail to provide help or brand them as hysterical, neurotic or misguided.

"Thus . . . we have a vastly informed public at the same time the bulk of the standard medical profession fails to recognize the yeast syndrome as a bona fide condition . . . It is a complex of conditions, a disease process that may be a primary or secondary disorder. The yeast overgrowth complex, silent or evident, usually manifests itself in the gastrointestinal tract. It is one of those conditions . . . that often quietly produces over the years a load of unwanted chemicals, toxins, macromolecules or partially digested foods that, in turn, adversely impact the liver and other target organs . . . All this usually occurs gradually over months, years, even decades of life . . .

"As one studies the yeast connection, one is struck by the rampant side effects of the chemical, dietary and antibiotic assaults made upon us since the industrial revolution, the introduction of processed foods and the medical profession's love affair with antibiotics. Lest I come across as a radical nihilist in human affairs, let me assert that the march of progress of civilization has at the same time provided us with amazing benefits. Yet I recognize too the enormous price that each of us has paid and is paying for the advances of civilization. Part of that price is the yeast complex."[2]

REFERENCES

1. Crook, W.G., *The Yeast Connection,* Professional Books, Jackson, TN and Vintage Books, New York, NY, 1986.
2. Wunderlich, R.C., *The Candida-Yeast Syndrome,* A Keats Good Health Guide, Keats Publishing, 1997.

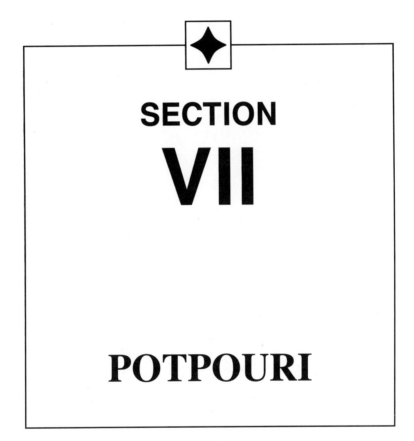

SECTION
VII

POTPOURI

Potpourri

Anemia

Many tired people are taking iron supplements which they do not need. Here are two of the reasons.

- ✦ They look pale and show dark circles under their eyes (common characteristics of the allergic person) even though they are not anemic.
- ✦ They have read or heard advertisements which suggest that they may have "tired" blood.

Although anemia may occur in men or women who are malnourished, suffer from a chronic infection or a bleeding peptic ulcer, or women who lose an excessive amount of blood through menstruation, *supplemental iron should not be taken if it is not needed*.

To obtain more information, I consulted my friend Elmer Cranton, M.D., a graduate of Harvard Medical School, who said,

> "Iron is so potentially dangerous that I recommend blood testing before prescribing it for anyone. Too much iron can shorten a person's life. . . If you just do a complete blood count—the hemoglobin hematocrit will sometimes come up below the reference range. It looks like they're iron deficient, but they are often not. Before you ever give iron, you should measure the serum iron and the iron binding capacity. Any laboratory who carries out these two tests will give you the percent saturation. The normal range is somewhere between 15 and 50%. I prefer a level under 25%. Ferritin above 12, but less than 100 is a cross check."

Why does taking unneeded iron supplements cause trouble? Many foods are already fortified with supplemental iron. Problems which develop from excessive iron intake may have to do with free radicals and iron appears to increase free radical damage, speeding the aging depression.

Herbal Remedy for Fibromyalgia

According to a report in the May 2000 issue of *Phytotherapy Research,* dietary supplementation with the alga *Chlorella pyrenoidosa* may relieve symptoms of fibromyalgia in some patients. The article cited studies by researchers at the Medical College of Virginia in Richmond. The researchers stated that the results of their findings in a study on 18 fibromyalgia patients suggest that the addition of *Chlorella* to the diet produced a significant reduction in their pain after only two months. They also said that their findings justify a larger clinical trial of *Chlorella* supplementation.* (This investigation was funded by a company producing the supplement used in the study.)

Energize Your Life

In her article in *Let's Live* magazine entitled "Best Ways to Energize Your Life," Lisa Turner gave readers a number of suggestions, including those made by JoHannah Reiley, N.D., a Boulder, Colorado naturopath and acupuncturist. Here are some of them.

> "Eat more protein and cut down on simple carbohydrates . . . Build your power lunch around veggies, raw or cooked, with lean meat, fish or beans . . . Break the caffeine habit. . . Wind down. An hour before bedtime start slowing down. Do gentle stretches and take a hot bath, make a cup of chamomile tea—whatever works for you to calm your body and quiet your mind . . .

Phytotherapy Research, 2000; 14:167-173.

"Cut down on cell phone use. If possible turn off fluorescent lights at work and use a desk lamp or standing lamp instead. Be a water snob. Always drink bottled or purified water and drink it at comfortable temperature. Meditate under a tree, head for the hills for an energetic hike, paint or draw outside on your lunch break."

In her concluding paragraph headed "The Bottom Line," Turner said,

"Ask yourself if you're having fun and creating meaning in your life. Focus on activities that move your soul and allow your source of energy to come from deeper within. 'Remember what life is about,' Reiley says. 'We're here to live and love and be happy. It's really just that simple.'"*

Fibromyalgia Syndrome (FMS)

In discussing this syndrome in *The Yeast Connection and the Woman*, I said,

"At several conferences on chronic fatigue syndrome professionals who discussed this disorder expressed varying points of view and different treatments were recommended. *The general consensus seemed to be that FM and chronic fatigue syndrome were closely related—if not the same disorder.*

"In discussing terminology, Kristen Thorson, publisher, *Fibromyalgia Network,* said Dr. Dan Goldenberg made the following comments during an interview in 1989. 'What you call it [FMS or CFIDS] depends on the eyes of the beholder. I'm convinced that Dr. Goldenberg was correct. FMS could be another name for CFIDS . . . or vice versa, depending on which diagnosis you happen to have.'"[1]

To learn more about FMS I consulted a number of experienced physicians, including Jorge Flechas, M.D., of Hender-

*Let's Live, November 1999, pp. 33–37.

sonville, North Carolina, who had provided me with information I included in several of my books. To obtain an update on his observations I called him in May 2000 and he told me about a number of therapies he had found effective. Here are brief excerpts from the extensive message on his web page www.fibromyhelp.com. In "A Message to the Health Practitioner," he said,

> "In the past eight years of working with fibromyalgia (FM) patients, I've concentrated on treatments that are as natural as possible, listening to my patients for possible solutions. I've tried herbs, amino acids and natural nutrients to relieve their pain."[2]

In his discussion he described his experiences using oxytocin in helping his patients with fibromyalgia, including those with cold hands, cold feet and headache.

On other parts of his web page, Dr. Flechas discussed the observations of Michael J. Rosner, M.D., FACS, FCCM, who has found that "there's a subset of patients with the diagnosis of Chronic Fatigue Immune Deficiency Syndrome or Fibromyalgia Syndrome who suffer from some element of craniovertebral compression." Dr. Rosner found that some of these patients could be relieved by surgery.[3]

Another therapy Dr. Flechas has used for many years in helping relieve FM pain is a product called Super Malic. The original malic acid/magnesium combination was developed by Optimox Corporation. Here are excerpts about this product from Dr. Flechas' web page.

> "The Super Malic® Plus daily nutritional program is a malic acid/magnesium-emphasized dietary program, which consists of dietary guidelines for consumption of foods rich in malic acid and magnesium; limitation of foods that block the absorption, that interfere with the utilization and that increase the

loss of magnesium; and Super Malic® Plus supplementation. . . For more information write to Optimox Corporation, P.O. Box 3378, Torrance, CA 90510-3378. Or call toll free 800-223-1601."[4]

Low Standing Blood Pressure and Chronic Fatigue

People with chronic fatigue syndrome (CFS) often show low blood pressure readings, especially after standing from a sitting position. A New York state study found that 15 CFS patients had significantly lower ($p < 0.001$) systolic (heart pumping) and diastolic (heart filling) blood pressure than 15 health-matched controls. Standing heart rates were significantly increased in the CFS patients ($p < 0.01$).

When 11 of these patients wore Military Anti Shock Trousers (MAST), which increased blood pressure on their legs and moved blood up to the brain, 10 patients (91%) reported improvement of their CFS symptoms.

In addition, red blood cell volume was significantly decreased in plasma and norepinephrine levels were significantly higher in the CFS patients.

Low blood pressure, especially in the brain, can cause fatigue and lack of concentration. Another study published in JAMA (1985; 274:961–7) noted that many CFS patients with low pressure reported reduction in symptoms when given a diet high in water and sodium. (emphasis added)*

Miracles

In his book *Miracles Do Happen,* C. Norman Shealy, M.D., a physician with impeccable personal and academic credentials said,

---

*Stretten, David, et al., "The Roles of Orthostatic Hypotension, Orthostatic Tachycardia, and Subnormal Erthyrocyte Volume in the Pathogenesis of Chronic Fatigue Syndrome, *American Journal of Medical Science,* July 2000; 320(1):1–8.

"Throughout medical history most illnesses have been treated with 'folk medicine.' Indeed, until the 1940s individuals were often better served if they avoided physicians or hospitals. Then the explosion of modern technological medicine began, with introduction of a never-ending array of diagnostic and therapeutic miracles: antibiotics, tranquilizers, remarkably complex surgery, CT scans, MRI and so on. These changes have given us the most successful medical system in history—for treatment of acute illness. Unfortunately, the glamour of these innovations have obscured the lack of attention to chronic illness . . .

"A vast majority of illnesses are still treated not by physicians but in the folk and alternative domain. A landmark article in the *New England Journal of Medicine* proved that Americans made more visits to alternative practitioners than they made to primary physicians . . . In the past 25 years I've lectured to many thousands of Americans eager for information on self care. Trained at the Massachusetts General Hospital in neurosurgery, I soon realized that drugs and surgery are inappropriate in the management of chronic pain . . .

"I consider any event or experience that transcends expectation, logic, or 'facts' as we believe them, and that provides a numinous life change, to be a *miracle*. . . As Sir William Osler, the Father of American Medicine said almost 100 years ago: 'Far more important than what the physician does is the patient's belief and the physician's belief in what the physician does.'

". . . Conventional medicine has exhausted our belief in the effectiveness of drugs and surgery. Although the conventional approach promises miraculous cures, it often provides only temporary treatment of symptoms and side effects. Fortunately, many alternatives still hold the potential for producing personal miracles.

"I first became aware of miracles a quarter century ago. Prior to that time, even though miracles occurred regularly, I never noticed them. Actually, they occur in all of our lives—

almost often enough to cease being miracles . . . we often don't recognize or acknowledge them . . .

"To a large extent, all the current interest in alternative medicine is a long-delayed acknowledgment by the public that conventional, allopathic medicine has ignored the most important aspect of healing: the untapped miracle of the individual's personal will, intuition and heart. When will, intuition, and heart are united, even for a few moments, miracles occur."[5]

MSG—A Food Additive Which Can Cause Dangerous Reactions

The term MSG stands for a processed free glutamic acid which causes nervous system and other reactions in sensitive people. Food products that always contain MSG include monosodium glutamate, textured protein, hydrolyzed protein and yeast extract. There are also over two dozen foods which often contain MSG (or create MSG during processing) including soy sauce, bouillon, natural beef flavoring, soy protein isolate and anything fermented.

According to a comprehensive article in the Spring 2000 issue of *NOHA News,** which featured the observations of Mr. Jack Samuels and NOHA board member, Adrienne Samuels, Ph.D.,[†]

> "Some people are sensitive to minute amounts of free glutamic acid. For others a larger dose or more than one dose is required to elicit reactions, which can be either immediate or delayed. In all cases, babies and small children are most vulnerable. What should we do?

NOHA News is published quarterly by Nutritional Optimal Health Association, a nonprofit organization. For a copy of the newsletter containing the article, send $3.00 to NOHA, P.O. Box 386, Winnetka, IL 60093 and request NOHA News for Spring 2000.

†For more information contact Jack and Andrienne Samuels at the Truth in Labeling Campaign, P.O. Box 2532, Darien, IL 60561; adandjack@aol.com; or www.truthin labeling.org.

(1) For ourselves individually, we need to consume truly natural, unfermented, unadulterated, unprocessed protein.

(2) For everyone everywhere, we need to communicate through our friends and relatives, our local newspapers, over the internet, and to our congresspersons and senators the facts about the deceptive research and the misleading food labeling.

"When the word spreads and the public demands food without neurotoxic free glutamic acid, then our lives can be dramatically improved and we can be free from this often hidden source of suffering.

Inhaled Corticosteroids and Oral Candidiasis

According to a report in the *Journal of Clinical Epidemiology,* oral candidiasis (OC) is a frequent side effect of inhaled corticosteroids (iCSTs). In this report researchers from the University of Montreal, Montreal, Quebec, Canada, studied the medical records of 27,000 seniors using antiasthma medications.

"The three year occurrence for OC was 7%. Increased risk for a first occurrence of OC was significantly associated with higher doses of iCST, increased length of iCST exposure, use of antibiotics . . . and concurrent use of oral steroids and diabetes medications. The occurrence of OC is relatively high. Knowledge of factors leading to increased risk could facilitate the targetting of patients who need timely intervention, under conditions of normal use."[6]

Quercetin

This is one of a group of plant pharmaceuticals called flavonoids. According to nutritional authority Michael Murray, N.D., flavonoids were discovered by Nobel Prize winner Albert St. Györgi while he was carrying out research on vitamin C. Initially this Hungarian scientist termed his discovery vitamin P, but this designation was later abandoned.

Although flavonoids are often referred to as "semi-essential" nutrients, apparently they're as important in human nutrition as essential vitamins and minerals. Other flavonoids include citrus bioflavonoids, grape seed extract and green tea polythenols. According to Murray,

> "Flavonoids as a group possess significant antiviral activity, quercetin having the greatest antiviral activity . . . *In vitro* it seems to inhibit both viral replication and infectivity. *In vivo* studies in animals have also shown quercetin to inhibit viral infections. . . Quercetin is consistently the most active of the flavonoids in experimental studies and many medicinal plants owe much of their activity to their high quercetin content. . . Based largely on *in vitro* studies quercetin appears indicated in virtually all inflammatory and allergic conditions (including asthma, hay fever, rheumatoid arthritis and lupus and in diabetes and cancer)."[7]

Murray acknowledged, however, that one of the shortcomings about claims for quercetin is a lack of clinical studies and the questionable quercetin absorption. According to Murray the recommended dose for quercetin is 200–400 mg, twenty minutes before meals, three times a day.

Sublingual Immunotherapy

In the early 1970s, several of my colleagues in the Society for Clinical Ecology (present name: American Academy of Environmental Medicine—AAEM) told me that sublingual doses of allergy extracts helped them in testing and treating their patients. I was skeptical, and so were my pediatric associates in the Jackson, Tennessee, Children's Clinic.

I received even more information from my allergy technician, the late Nell Sellers, who spent the day with Dr. Guy Pfeiffer in his office in Mattoon, Illinois. When she returned she said, *"I talked to many people who said that sublingual extracts were amazingly effective in relieving their symptoms caused by inhalant and food sensitivities."*

Based on Nell's report, I slowly began to use these extracts in my own allergy practice and I was delighted when this therapy helped many of my patients. My pediatric practice partners continued to be skeptical and felt that my patients' improvement was a placebo reaction.

My colleagues in major allergy organizations were even more skeptical, and called this type of testing and treatment "witchcraft." Nevertheless, a growing number of AAEM members found that allergy extracts administered sublingually were as effective as those given by injection.

Then, in 1999, I was delighted to read an article[8] and an editorial on sublingual immunotherapy in the *Journal of Allergy and Clinical Immunology*. Here are excerpts from the editorial.

"Few things incite more argument among allergists than specific allergen immunotherapy. For some specific immunotherapy (SIT) is the treatment that defines our speciality. For others, it is a relic of 19th Century clinical practice that we should discard in favor of modern pharmacotherapy. The evidence for SIT was mostly gathered long before the modern era of double-blind, placebo-control randomized trials.

"Several recent studies have reported beneficial effects of sublingual immunotherapy on symptoms of allergic rhinitis. . . In this month's issue of the *Journal,* LaRosa, et al., report on a 2-year study of sublingual immunotherapy in children age 6–14 years with allergic rhinoconjunctivitis. . . This study provides encouragement for those interested in this novel route of administration, provides some useful evidences of efficacy in younger patients. . . Currently, sublingual immunotherapy continues to look promising, but further studies are needed."[9]

My Comments: Although the recent article and editorial provide support for sublingual immunotherapy, the subject may remain controversial for many reasons. Here's one of them. The dose of antigens (allergens) in the European study were larger than the "neutralizing" doses which most of my colleagues and I used in treating our patients.

Twenty-one articles describing sublingual immunotherapy have been published in the medical literature. Included is an article by David L. Morris, M.D., entitled "Treatment of Respiratory Disease with Ultra-Small Doses of Antigens." (Vol. 28, pp. 494–500, October 1970.) To obtain a list of the references write to the American Academy of Environmental Medicine, 7701 E. Kellogg, Suite 625, Wichita, KS 67207.

REFERENCES

1. Crook, W.G., *The Yeast Connection and the Woman*, Professional Books, Jackson, TN, 1995/1998, pp. 188–189.
2. Flechas, J., www.fibromyhelp.com/todoctors.html.
3. Flechas, J., www.fibromyhelp.com/Rosnerneck.html.
4. Flechas, J., www.fibromyhelp.com/treatments.html.
5. Shealy, C.N., *Miracles Do Happen*, Element Books, Inc., P.O. Box 830, Rockport, MA 01966, 1995, pp. 3–9.
6. Kennedy, W.A., et al., "Occurrence and risk factors of oral candidiasis treated with oral antifungals in seniors using inhaled steroids," *Journal of Clinical Epidemiology*, 53(2000) 696–701.
7. Murray, M., *Encyclopedia of Nutritional Supplements*, Primer Publishing, Rockland, CA, 1996, pp. 320–330.
8. LaRosa, M., et al., "Double-blind placebo-controlled evaluation of sublingual-swallow immunotherapy with standardized *Parietaria judaica* extract in children with allergic rhinoconjunctivitis," *Journal of Allergy and Clinical Immunology*, 1999; 104:425–32.
9. Frew, A.J., White, P.J. and Smith, H.E., "Sublingual Immunotherapy," *Journal of Allergy and Clinical Immunology*, 1999; 104:267–270.

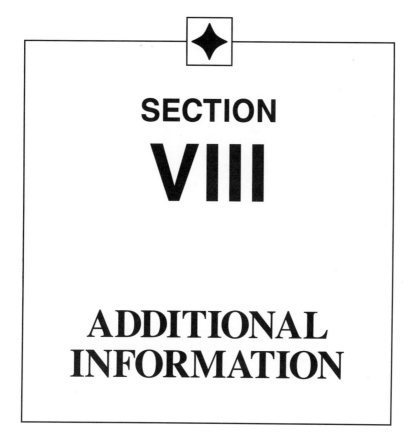

SECTION

VIII

ADDITIONAL
INFORMATION

Questionnaire

Candida Questionnaire
and Score Sheet

If you'd like to know if your health problems are yeast-connected, take this comprehensive questionnaire.

Questions in Section A focus on your medical history—factors that promote the growth of *Candida albicans* and that frequently are found in people with yeast-related health problems.

In Section B you'll find a list of 23 symptoms that are often present in patients with yeast-related health problems. Section C consists of 33 other symptoms that are sometimes seen in people with yeast-related problems—yet they also may be found in people with other disorders.

Filling out and scoring this questionnaire should help you and your physician evaluate the possible role *Candida albicans* contributes to your health problems. Yet, it will not provide an automatic "yes" or "no" answer.

Section A: History

	Point Score
1. Have you taken tetracyclines or other antibiotics for acne for 1 month (or longer)?	35
2. Have you at any time in your life taken broad-spectrum antibiotics or other antibacterial medication for respiratory, urinary or other infections for two months or longer, or in shorter courses four or more times in a one-year period?	35

Candida Questionnaire
and Score Sheet—*Cont'd.*

Section A: History—*Cont'd.*

	Point Score
3. Have you taken a broad-spectrum antibiotic drug—even in a single dose?	6
4. Have you, at any time in your life, been bothered by persistent prostatitis, vaginitis or other problems affecting your reproductive organs?	25
5. Are you bothered by memory or concentration problems—do you sometimes feel spaced out?	20
6. Do you feel "sick all over" yet, in spite of visits to many different physicians, the causes haven't been found?	20
7. Have you been pregnant . . . Two or more times? One time?	5 3
8. Have you taken birth control pills . . . For more than two years? For six months to two years?	15 8
9. Have you taken steroids orally, by injection or inhalation? For more than two weeks? For two weeks or less?	15 6
10. Does exposure to perfumes, insecticides, fabric shop odors and other chemicals provoke . . . Moderate to severe symptoms? Mild symptoms?	20 5
11. Does tobacco smoke *really* bother you?	10
12. Are your symptoms worse on damp, muggy days or in moldy places?	20

Point Score

13. Have you had athlete's foot, ring worm, "jock itch" or other chronic fungous infections of the skin or nails? Have such infections been . . .
    Severe or persistent?   20
    Mild to moderate?   10

14. Do you crave sugar?   10

TOTAL SCORE, Section A

Section B: Major Symptoms

For each of your symptoms, enter the appropriate figure in the Point Score column:

If a symptom is **occasional or mild** .... 3 points
If a symptom is **frequent and/or moderately severe** .... 6 points
If a symptom is **severe and/or disabling** .... 9 points

Add total score and record it at the end of this section.

Point Score

1. Fatigue or lethargy

2. Feeling of being "drained"

3. Depression or manic depression

4. Numbness, burning or tingling

5. Headache

6. Muscle aches

7. Muscle weakness or paralysis

8. Pain and/or swelling in joints

9. Abdominal pain

10. Constipation and/or diarrhea

11. Bloating, belching or intestinal gas

12. Troublesome vaginal burning, itching or discharge

Candida Questionnaire
and Score Sheet—*Cont'd.*

Section B: Major Symptoms—*Cont'd.*

Point Score

13. Prostatitis

14. Impotence

15. Loss of sexual desire or feeling

16. Endometriosis or infertility

17. Cramps and/or other menstrual irregularities

18. Premenstrual tension

19. Attacks of anxiety or crying

20. Cold hands or feet, low body temperature

21. Hypothyroidism

22. Shaking or irritable when hungry

23. Cystitis or interstitial cystitis

TOTAL SCORE, Section B

Section C: Other Symptoms

For each of your symptoms, enter the appropriate figure in the Point Score column:

If a symptom is **occasional or mild** .... 1 point
If a symptom is **frequent and/or moderately severe** .... 2 points
If a symptom is **severe and/or disabling** .... 3 points

Add total score and record it at the end of this section.

1. Drowsiness, including inappropriate drowsiness

2. Irritability

Point Score

3. Incoordination

4. Frequent mood swings

5. Insomnia

6. Dizziness/loss of balance

7. Pressure above ears . . . feeling of head swelling

8. Sinus problems . . . tenderness of cheekbones or forehead

9. Tendency to bruise easily

10. Eczema, itching eyes

11. Psoriasis

12. Chronic hives (urticaria)

13. Indigestion or heartburn

14. Sensitivity to milk, wheat, corn or other common foods

15. Mucus in stools

16. Rectal itching

17. Dry mouth or throat

18. Mouth rashes, including "white" tongue

19. Bad breath

20. Foot, hair or body odor not relieved by washing

21. Nasal congestion or postnasal drip

22. Nasal itching

23. Sore throat

24. Laryngitis, loss of voice

Candida Questionnaire
and Score Sheet—*Cont'd.*

Section C: Other Symptoms—*Cont'd.*

Point Score

25. Cough or recurrent bronchitis

26. Pain or tightness in chest

27. Wheezing or shortness of breath

28. Urinary frequency or urgency

29. Burning on urination

30. Spots in front of eyes or erratic vision

31. Burning or tearing eyes

32. Recurrent infections or fluid in ears

33. Ear pain or deafness

TOTAL SCORE, Section C

Total Score, Section A

Total Score, Section B

GRAND TOTAL SCORE

The Grand Total Score will help you and your physician decide if your health problems are yeast-connected. Scores in women will run higher, as seven items in the questionnaire apply exclusively to women, while only two apply exclusively to men.

Yeast-connected health problems are almost certainly present in women with scores **more than 180,** and in men with scores **more than 140.**

Yeast-connected health problems are probably present in women with scores **more than 120,** and in men with scores **more than 90.**

Yeast-connected health problems are possibly present in women with scores **more than 60,** and in men with scores **more than 40.**

With scores of less than 60 in women and 40 in men, yeasts are less apt to cause health problems.

International Health Foundation

International Health Foundation

After the publication of *The Yeast Connection* in 1983, I received tens of thousands of letters and phone calls from people seeking a physician to help them. To respond to this need, the International Health Foundation (IHF) was incorporated in Tennessee in 1985. The Internal Revenue Service granted the IHF non-profit, tax exempt status in 1986.

During the past 15 years, this foundation received more than 70,000 letters from people seeking a physician and other information. In response, IHF established a roster of physicians and sent people a list of physicians in their area who were interested in yeast-related disorders.

Although some people who wrote IHF were able to find a physician through the IHF lists, this approach has left much to be desired. Here are a few of the reasons. In spite of our persistent efforts, fewer than 800 physicians in the United States are listed on the IHF referral roster. Here are other limitations:

✦ Many physicians listed are so busy that the waiting period to obtain an appointment may be many months.
✦ The offices of physicians listed may be hundreds of miles from you.
✦ Physicians listed may not be a member of your health insurance plan.

Although you *may* be able to find help from a physician on the IHF list, *your personal physician may be your best option.* Here's a suggestion which many people who have written and called me have found effective.

If your personal physician is kind and caring, although skeptical of the relationship of yeast to your health problems, write her/him a letter and say,

> Thank you for the patience you've shown in listening to my complaints and for the help you've given me. Yet, in spite of a number of tests and therapies which I've received, I'm continuing to experience health problems that I feel may be yeast-related. Will you work with me?
>
> I realize that you may not believe that yeasts play a part in causing my symptoms. I can understand your point of view. *There is, however, new scientific support of the relationship of yeast to a number of chronic illnesses.*
>
> There are also reports of the effectiveness of nystatin, Diflucan, Lamisil, Sporanox and Nizoral in helping people with a diverse group of chronic illnesses.

In our efforts to respond to the people who write and call IHF seeking help for their own health problems or for their children's health problems, in 2000 IHF completed the following new publications:

1. A 36-page booklet for adults, *Information For You,* which includes information about diets, medications and a list of 800 health professionals who have expressed an interest in treating patients with yeast-related disorders.
2. A 76-page booklet, *Children's Health Problems.* In this booklet I discuss children with recurring ear disorders, fatigue, headache, respiratory complaints, "hidden" food allergies, ADHD, autism and/or other serious developmental problems.

Although I don't claim to possess a "quick fix" for any or all of these problems, information I acquired from many sources shows that they are often yeast-connected.

3. A 24-page booklet, *A Special Message to the Health Professional.* Included in this booklet is a discussion of the yeast controversy and reports from the mid and late 1990s which support the relationship of yeast infections to many chronic health disorders. These include: asthma, autism, chronic fatigue syndrome, endometriosis, fibromyalgia, headaches, interstitial cystitis, multiple sclerosis and psoriasis.

To obtain booklets 1 and 3 or 2 and 3, send a tax deductible donation of $25 to IHF, Box 3494, Jackson, TN 38303-3494. For all three booklets, send $35. *If you aren't pleased with the information in these booklets, your money will be refunded.*

You can also find additional information about Dr. Crook and the International Health Foundation on the Internet at www.candida-yeast.com. If you have questions, you may call Dr. Crook on the IHF hotline (901-660-7090) most Tuesdays between 12:45 and 2:15 P.M. Central time.

Other Sources of Information

Although you'll learn a lot from searching the Internet, books, magazines and newsletters will provide you with solid information you can read and re-read. Here are sources I've consulted in writing this book.

Books

Baker, Sidney and Baar, Karen, *The Circadian Prescription,* G. P. Putnam & Sons, New York, 2000.

Baker, Sidney, *Detoxification and Healing,* Keats Publishing, New Canaan, CT, 1997.

Carper, Jean, *Miracle Cures,* Harper Collins, New York, 1997.

Carrigan, Catherine, *Healing Depression: A Holistic Guide,* Marlowe and Company, New York, 1999.

Challem, Jack, *All About Vitamins,* Avery Publishing Group, Garden City, New York, 1988.

Colborn, Theo, Dumanoski, Dianne and Meyer, John P., *Our Stolen Future,* Plume/Penguin, New York, 1997.

Connolly, Pat and Associates of the Price-Pottenger Nutrition Foundation, *The Candida albicans Yeast-Free Cookbook,* Second edition, Keats Publishing, Los Angeles, CA, 1985, 2000.

Cranton, Elmer and Fryer, William, *Resetting the Clock—5 Anti-Aging Hormones That Are Revolutionizing The Quality and Length Of Life,* M. Evans and Company, New York, 1996. (Available by calling 800-337-9918)

Crook, William and Jones, Marge, *The Yeast Connection Cookbook,* Professional Books, Jackson, TN, 1989/1997.

Crook, William, *The Yeast Connection and the Woman*, Professional Books, Jackson, TN, 1995/1998.

Crook, William, *The Yeast Connection Handbook*, Professional Books, Jackson, TN, 1996/1998/2000.

Crook, William, *Nature's Own Candida Cure*, Canada, Alive Books, Vancouver, B.C., 2000.

Dossey, Larry, *Reinventing Medicine—Beyond Mind-Body to a New Era of Healing*, Harper, San Francisco, 1999.

Galland, Leo, *Power Healing*, Random House, New York, 1998.

Goldberg, Burton and editors of *Alternative Medicine Guide to Chronic Fatigue, Fibromyalgia and Environmental Illness*, Tiburon, CA, 1998.

Haas, Elson, *The False Fat Diet*, Ballentine Books, New York, 2000.

Haas Elson, *The Staying Healthy Shopper's Guide*, Celestial Arts, Berkeley, CA, 1999.

Hobbs, Christopher and Haas, Elson, *Vitamins for Dummies*, IDG Books Worldwide, Foster City, CA, 1999.

Hoffman, Ronald, *Tired All the Time*, Poseidon, New York, 1993.

Jacob, S.W., Lawrence, R.M. and Zucker, M., *The Miracle of MSM—The Natural Solution for Pain*, Berkley Books, New York, 1999.

Krimsky, Sheldon, *Hormonal Chaos*, Johns Hopkins University Press, Baltimore, MD, 2000.

Lawson, Lynn, *Staying Well in a Toxic World*, Lynnword Press, Evanston, IL, 1993.

Martin, Jeanne Marie with Rona Zoltan, *Complete Candida Yeast Guidebook*, Revised Second Edition, Prima Health, Roseville, CA, 2000.

Meyerowitz, Steve, *Power Juices Super Drinks*, Kensington Publishing Corp., New York, 2000.

Murray, Michael, *Encyclopedia of Nutritional Supplements,* Prima Publishing, Rocklin, CA, 1997.

Murray, Michael and Pizzorno, Joseph, *Encyclopedia of Natural Medicine,* Second edition, Prima Publishing, Rocklin, CA, 1997.

Peale, Norman Vincent, *Imaging—The Powerful Way to Change Your Life,* Guideposts, Carmel, NY, 1982.

Prevention editors, *Doctor's Book of Home Remedies for Preventing Disease,* Rodale Press, Emmaus, PA, 1999.

Rapp, Doris J., *Is This Your Child's World? How You Can Fix the Schools and Homes That Are Making Your Children Sick,* Bantam Books, New York, 1996.

Rea, William, *Chemical Sensitivity,* Volumes I—IV, CRC Press, Boca Raton, FL.

Rogers, S.A., *Tired or Toxic?,* Prestige Publishing, Syracuse, NY, 1990.

Rogers, S.A., *Depression: Cured At Last!,* Prestige Publishing, Syracuse, NY, 1998.

Rona, Zoltan P., *Return to the Joy of Health,* Alive Books, Burnaby, BC, Canada, 1995.

Sahley, Billie J., *Malic Acid and Magnesium for Fibromyalgia and Chronic Pain Syndrome,* 7th edition, Pain and Stress Publications, San Antonio, TX, 1999.

Schmidt, Michael, *Tired of Being Tired?,* Frog, Ltd., Berkeley, CA, 1995.

Schmidt, Michael, *Smart Fats—How Dietary Fats and Oils Affect Mental, Physical and Emotional Intelligence,* Frog, Ltd., Berkeley, CA, 1997. (Distributed by North Atlantic Books, P.O. Box 12327, Berkeley, CA 94712.)

Shealy, C. Norman, *Miracles Do Happen—A Physician's Experience with Alternative Medicine,* Element Books, Rockport, MA, 1995.

Sinatra, Stephen T., *The Co-Enzyme Q10 Phenomenon,* Lowell House, Los Angeles, CA, 1998.

Spreen, Allan N., *Nutritionally Incorrect,* Woodland Publishing, Pleasant Grove, UT, 1999.

Walker, Morton, *Olive Leaf Extract,* Kensington, New York, 1997.

Wittenberg, Janice S., *The Rebellious Body - Reclaiming your life from environmental illness or chronic fatigue syndrome,* Insight Books, Plenum Press, New York/London, 1996.

Wunderlich, Ray A., *The Candida Yeast Syndrome,* (booklet), Keats Publishing, New Canaan, CT, 1997.

Zand, Janet, Spreen, Allen and LaValle, James, *Smart Medicine for Healthier Living,* Avery Publishing Group, Garden City Park, NY, 1999.

Newsletters and Magazines

Alive—Canadian Journal of Health and Nutrition, published 11 times a year. 7436 Fraser Park Dr., Burnaby, B.C., Canada, V5J 5B9. $24.50.

Better Nutrition for Today's Living, published monthly by Communication Channels, Inc., 6151 Powers Ferry Rd., N.W., Atlanta, GA 30339. Available in most health food stores (404-955-2500).

Bottom Line Health, 55 Railroad Avenue, Greenwich, CT 06836-2614. Published monthly. $49/year.

Canary News, Newsletter of the Chicago area Environmental Illness/Multiple Chemical Sensitivities (EI/MSC) Support Group, 1404 Judson Ave., Evanston, IL 60201. $15/year.

CFIDS Chronicle, the bi-monthly publication of the Chronic Fatigue and Immune Dysfunction Syndrome Association of America, P.O. Box 220398, Charlotte, NC 28222-0398. Fax: 704-365-9755, 800-442-3437. www.cfids.org.

Clinical Pearls News, A Health Letter on Current Research in Nutrition and Preventive Medicine published by I. T. Services, 3302 Alta Arden #2, Sacramento, CA 95825. (916-483-1085). $109/year, 12 issues.

Delicious! Magazine, 1301 Spruce St., Boulder, CO 80302 (303-939-8440).

Dr. Christiane Northrup's *Health Wisdom for Women,* published monthly by Phillips Publishing Company, Inc., 7811 Montrose Road, Potomac, MD 20854 (301-340-2100).

Dr. Julian Whitaker's *Health & Healing—Tomorrow's Medicine Today,* published monthly by Phillips Publishing Company, Inc., 7811 Montrose Rd., Potomac, MD 20854 (301-340-2100). $39/year.

Dr. Jonathan Wright's *Nutrition and Healing,* published monthly by Agora South, L.L.C., 819 N. Charles St., Baltimore, MD 21201 (410-223-2611). $74/year.

Fibromyalgia Network, A newsletter for people with Fibromyalgia Syndrome/Chronic Fatigue Syndrome, P.O. Box 31750, Tucson, AZ 85751-1750. 800-853-2929; Fax: 520-290-5550.www.fmnetnews.com. $25/year, 4 issues.

Let's Live, America's foremost health and preventive magazine, 444 N. Larchmont Blvd., Los Angeles, CA 90004. Published monthly. $19.95/year.

Lifeline, Quarterly newsletter of the Wisconsin Chronic Fatigue Association, Inc., 1001 W. Main St., Sun Prairie, WI 53590. (608-834-1001). www.wicfs.me.org. $20/year, 4 issues.

NOHA News, published by Nutrition for Optimal Health (NOHA), P. O. Box 380, Winnetka, IL 60093. $8/year, published quarterly.

Nutrition Action Healthletter, CSPI, 1875 Connecticut Ave. N.W., Washington, D.C. 20009. $24/yr., 10 issues.

Nutrition Science News, Published monthly by New Hope Communications, Inc., 1301 Spruce St., Boulder, CO 80302-4832. $39/year.

Sully's Living Without—a lifestyle guide to achieving better health. P.O. Box 132, Clarendon Hills, IL 60514-0132. $16/ yr., published quarterly.

The Townsend Letter for Doctors and Patients, 911 Tyler St., Port Townsend, WA 98366-6541 (360-385-6021). $49/10 issues yearly.

Pharmacies

Oral preparations of sugar-free, dye-free nystatin powder and capsules can be obtained on prescription from these pharmacies. So can most of the nonprescription agents and nutritional supplements discussed in this book.

The Apothecary, Bethesda, MD 20814, 800-869-9159, Fax: 301-493-4671.

Bio Tech Pharmacy,* Fayetteville, AR, 72702, 800-345-1199, Fax: 501-443-5643

College Pharmacy, Colorado Springs, CO, 80903, 800-888-9356, Fax: 800-556-5893.

Freeda Pharmacy, New York, NY, 10017 800-777-3737, Fax: 212-685-7297.

Hopewell Pharmacy and Compounding, Hopewell, NJ 08525, 800-792-6670, Fax: 800-417-3864.

Medical Towers Pharmacy, Birmingham, AL 35205, 800-378-7877 or 205-933-7381.

N.E.E.D.S., Syracuse, NY 13209, 800-634-1380, Fax: 315-488-6336.

Wellness Health and Pharmaceuticals, Birmingham, AL 35209, 800-227-2627, Fax: 800-369-0302.

Willner Chemist, New York, NY 10017, 800-633-1106, Fax: 212-682-6192.

_____

*Wholesale supplier to other pharmacies.

Women's International Pharmacy, 5708 Monona Dr., Madison,
WI 53716-3152, 800-279-5708, Fax: 800-279-8011.

Nutritional Supplements

Vitamins/minerals, antioxidants and many of the other products discussed in this book are available in health food stores and
from other sources including:

CFIDS & FM Health Resource, 805-564-3064, www.immune
support.com
Douglas Laboratories, 800-245-4440 or 888-368-4522;
www.douglaslabs.com; e-mail: nutrition@douglaslabs.com
Swanson Health Products, 800-437-4148, www.swanson
vitamins.com

Internet Sources

www.candida-yeast.com
www.greatplainslaboratory.com
www.imbris/~mastent/
www.candidapage.com
www.savorypalate.com
www.autism.com/ari
www.nlci.com/nutrition
www.cssa-inc.org
www.hhi.org
www.drmagaziner.com
www.drcranton.com
www.wellnesshealth.com
www.cfs-recovery.org
www.parentsofallergicchildren.org
www.needs.com
www.alternativementalhealth.com
www.sbakermd.com
www.mdheal.org
www.geocities.com/HotSprings/2125/

Index

AAL Reference Laboratory, tests for yeast-related disorders, 290
Abdominal pain, 43, 53
Abraham, Guy, 105–106
Actimel, 222–223
Action Against Allergy (AAA), 71
acupuncture, 245–248
adenosine triphosphate (ATP), 331–332
ADHD. *See* attention deficit hyperactivity disorder
adrenal hormones: cortisol, 249–251; DHEA, 251–255
airborne allergens, 257–260
Alive, 66
Alka Seltzer Gold, 206
Allergic Tension-Fatigue Syndrome, 29, 31, 32
allergies, 208–209; and CFS, 9; and molds, 257–260; and sublingual immunotherapy, 353–355. *See also* food allergies and sensitivities
alpha lipoic acid (ALA), 229, 235–236
alternative medicine, 42, 226, 320–321, 350
amaranth, 65, 200
American Academy of Allergy, Asthma and Immunology, 24, 162
American Academy of Environmental Medicine, 68, 69, 353, 355
American Association of Chronic Fatigue Syndrome (AACFS), 16
American College of Allergy, Asthma and Immunology, 24, 162
American Family Physician, 308
American Lung Association, 260
American Medical Association, 24
amphotericin B (Fungizone),12, 172
Annals of Allergy, 258
Annals of Internal Medicine, 16

anemia, 345–346
antibiotics, 303–304; and candida-related health problems, 5, 37, 44, 51–52, 53–54, 74, 144, 156–157, 304, 318–319; and chronic fatigue syndrome, 39; and probiotics, 217, 224, 304
antioxidants, 228–230
antiyeast agents (nonprescription), 182–194; citrus seed extract, 182, 190–191; garlic, 188–189, 192, 193; Kolorex, 183, 185–186; olive leaf extract (OLE), 183–185, 192; oregano, 183, 190; ParaCan, 191; Tanalbit, 182, 189–190, 192, 193; undecylenic acid, 183, 186–188
antiyeast medications (prescription). *See* Diflucan; Lamisil; Nizoral; nystatin; Sporanox
Arem, Ridha, 123
Armour thyroid medication, 122
Ashford, Nicholas, 148–150
aspartame, 64
asthma, 167–168, 180; and oral candidiasis, 352
Atkins, Robert, 96, 131–132
attention deficit hyperactivity disorder (ADHD), 22–23, 87, 195
autism, 94, 168

back pain, acupuncture for, 245, 248
bacteria, friendly, 92–94
Bahna, Sami, 195, 216
Baker, Sidney M., 6–7, 11, 97–98, 103, 198–199, 229–230, 251, 297–298, 306
Ballweg, Mary Lou, 151
Barkley, Russell H., 22
barley grass, 236

About the Author

William G. Crook, M.D., received his medical education and training at the University of Virginia, the Pennsylvania Hospital, Vanderbilt and Johns Hopkins. He is a fellow of the American Academy of Pediatrics, the American College of Allergy and Immunology and the American Academy of Environmental Medicine. He is a member of the American Medical Association, the American Academy of Allergy and Immunology, Alpha Omega Alpha and other medical organizations.

Dr. Crook is the author of 13 previous books and numerous reports in the medical and lay literature. For fifteen years he wrote a nationally syndicated health column, "Child Care" (*General Features* and the *Los Angeles Times* Syndicates).

Various of his publications have been translated into French, German, Japanese and Norwegian.

The Yeast Connection Handbook is the fifth in his series of books which deal with the relationship of *Candida albicans* to many puzzling health disorders. The titles include *The Yeast Connection, The Yeast Connection Cookbook, Chronic Fatigue Syndrome and the Yeast Connection,* and *The Yeast Connection and the Woman.*

Dr. Crook has been a popular guest on local, regional, national and international television and radio programs, including Oprah Winfrey, Sally Jessy Raphael, Regis Philbin, The 700 Club, Good Morning Australia, TV Ontario and the BBC.

He has addressed professional and lay groups in 39 states, all Canadian provinces, Australia, England, Italy, Mexico, The

Netherlands, New Zealand and Venezuela. And he has served as a visiting professor at Ohio State University, and the Universities of California (San Francisco) and Saskatchewan.

Dr. Crook lives in Jackson, Tennessee, with his wife, Betsy. They have three daughters and four grandchildren. His interests include helping people, golf, bridge, oil painting and travel.